Health Care Alliances and Conversions

James R. Schwartz and
H. Chester Horn, Jr.

Foreword by Linda Miller

Health Care Alliances and Conversions

A Handbook for Nonprofit Directors and Trustees

Jossey-Bass Publishers
San Francisco

Jossey-Bass books and products are available through most bookstores. To contact Jossey-Bass directly, call (888) 378-2537, fax to (800) 605-2665, or visit our website at www.josseybass.com.

Substantial discounts on bulk quantities of Jossey-Bass books are available to corporations, professional associations, and other organizations. For details and discount information, contact the special sales department at Jossey-Bass.

 Manufactured in the United States of America on Lyons Falls Turin Book. This paper is acid-free and 100 percent totally chlorine-free.

Library of Congress Cataloging-in-Publication Data

Schwartz, James R., 1946-
    Health care alliances and conversions: a handbook for nonprofit trustees / James R. Schwartz and H. Chester Horn, Jr.; foreword by Linda Miller. — 1st ed.
      p. cm.
    Includes index.
    ISBN 0-7879-4177-8 (acid-free paper)
    1. Health facilities—Law and legislation—United States.   2. Strategic alliances (Business)—Law and legislation—United States.   3. Hospital mergers—United States.
4. Hospital trustees—Legal status, laws, etc.—United States.   5. Charitable uses, trusts, and foundations—United States.   I. Horn, H. Chester, 1947–   II. Title.
KF3825 .S38 1999
344.73'03211—ddc21   98-40155

FIRST EDITION
HB Printing   10 9 8 7 6 5 4 3 2 1

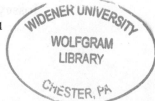

Contents

Acknowledgments

We would like to thank a number of people. First and foremost, we need to express our deep appreciation to Linda Miller, without whose support, encouragement, advice, and friendship this book might never have come into being. We would also like to thank Phil Isenberg; not only did he give us tremendous ideas on how to make the book better, but, as chair of the Judiciary Committee of the California Assembly, he authored the best hospital conversion law in the country and made it easy for us to do our job in protecting the interests of the people of California in these types of transactions. We would also like to thank Bud Lee for his excellent suggestions on how to make this book readable and helpful; we used them all.

Finally, and most important, one of us in particular would like to give special thanks to Kathy Horn for her support and patience during the writing of the book. It took far longer than we anticipated, and he owes you big-time for doing more than your fair share in caring for the Horn children, Margeaux, Danielle, Brooks, and Sasha.

This book was supported by the Volunteer Trustees
Foundation for Research and Education and the Commonwealth
Fund, a New York City–based private independent foundation.
Any views presented here are those of the authors and not
necessarily those of the Volunteer Trustees Foundation or the
Commonwealth Fund, its directors, officers, or staff.

The Authors

James R. Schwartz is a Deputy Attorney General with the California Attorney General's Office. For the past three years, Mr. Schwartz has had primary responsibility for overseeing all conversions of nonprofit hospitals within the State of California. In addition, he has been responsible for the review of numerous nonprofit to for-profit transactions. Described by California Attorney General Dan Lungren as the leading public sector professional in this area and by *California Medicine Magazine* as "the state's top expert on conversions," Mr. Schwartz has been responsible during this period for the review of fifteen separate transactions, involving sixteen acute care hospitals and additional HMOs, MSOs, and other ancillary businesses with an aggregate value in excess of $2 billion.

Mr. Schwartz is the author of the California Attorney General's Review Protocol for Ownership or Control Transfers of Non-Profit Health Facilities and was the principal drafter of the California law governing non-profit hospital sales (AB 3101-Isenberg).

In addition, he has written and spoken extensively on the subject of non-profit hospital conversions. His article, "The California Model" on nonprofit hospital conversions appeared in the March/April 1997 issue of *Health Affairs*; his article "Sales and other Transfers of Non-Profit Health Facilities: The Role of the Attorney General's Office in Reviewing and Approving These

Transactions" appeared in the Spring 1997 issue of *California Health Law News*; and his article (co-authored) "Deal Makers-Deal Breakers" appeared in the September 5, 1997 issue of *Hospitals and Health Networks*.

Previously, Mr. Schwartz headed a fourteen-person task force of attorneys, auditors, and investigators in a gubernatorial-requested probe of fraud in state-funded health care programs and was the supervising attorney for the principal litigation section of the Attorney General's office in San Francisco. As a charitable trust litigator specializing in officer-director liability cases, Mr. Schwartz has obtained over a half-dozen multi-million dollar recoveries in breach-of-trust cases involving universities, law schools, hospitals, and foundations. He is the recipient of the California Attorney General's Award for Excellence in Legal Services. Mr. Schwartz is a graduate of the Boalt Hall School of Law at the University of California, Berkeley.

H. Chester Horn, Jr. is a Deputy Attorney General in the Charitable Trusts Section of the California Attorney General's office. He has reviewed dozens of transfers of nonprofit hospital assets for the California Attorney General. Those transfers include nonprofit transactions as well as sales or joint ventures between nonprofit and for-profit entitites. Among the latter, Mr. Horn was responsible for reviewing the joint venture between the Riverside Community Hospital and Columbia/HCA, the sale of the three hospital systems of United Western Medical Centers to OrNda, the sale of the Rancho Murrietta Sharp Hospital to Tenet, and the sale and restructuring of Satellite Dialysis Centers, Inc. He also participated in the reviews of the proposed transactions involving the Sharp Hospital system in San Diego, California, the Centinela Valley Hospital in Los Angeles, California, the Desert Hospital in Indian Wells, California, and the Queen of Angels/Hollywood Presbyterian Medical Center in Los Angeles, California. Mr. Horn drafted the regulations implementing California's new hospital sale review statute, A.B. 3101, and has spoken extensively on nonprofit asset sales.

Prior to joining the Charitable Trusts section, Mr. Horn was assigned to the Antitrust Section of the California Department of Justice. While there, Mr. Horn successfully tried the two largest merger cases in the history of the office. In a case that successfully blocked a proposed merger of two of the largest supermarket chains in California, Mr. Horn argued before the United States Supreme Court establishing the right of state Attorneys General to dissolve mergers that violate federal antitrust laws. He also blocked the proposed merger between two of the three largest investor-owned electric utilities in California.

Mr. Horn has written extensively on mergers and acquisitions. He co-authored *Deal Makers, Deal Breakers*, Hospital and Health Networks, September 5, 1997. He also wrote: *The States' View of Regional and National Mergers*, 58 Antitrust Law Journal 233 (1989); *California v. American Stores: Some Thoughts About The Future For State Merger Enforcement Programs*, 18 NAAG *Antitrust Report*, No. 3, 1 (April-May Issue); *Some Suggestions for Confronting the Brave New World of Antitrust Federalism*, 36 *Antitrust Bulletin*, No. 4, at 821 (Winter, 1991); *Bank Mergers: A Unique Role for State Antitrust Enforcers?* No. 13 International Merger Law (Sept., 1991).

Mr. Horn lives in Malibu, California, with his wife, Kathy, and four children, Margeaux, Danielle, Brooks and Sasha. Mr. Horn is a graduate of the University of California at Santa Barbara and the U.C.L.A. School of Law.

Foreword

Linda Miller, President,
Volunteer Trustees Foundation
for Research and Education

The U.S. health care system is in upheaval, and perhaps no activity is more indicative of the depth of change underway than the selling of not-for-profit hospitals to for-profit companies. Community hospitals are on the block: religious hospitals, teaching hospitals, urban and rural hospitals, large and small hospitals; hospitals that have decades of tenure in our communities, that have been run by community boards, and that have been organized as nonprofits specifically to serve the community as a whole, rich and poor members of it alike.

The selling off of not-for-profit hospital assets has taken place in hundreds of communities, triggering the largest redeployment of charitable assets in the nation's history. Whether these sales are good for the communities or their health care systems, only time will tell. But how these decisions get made and how the sales are structured are issues for the present. Literally billions of health care dollars once invested in community-owned, not-for-profit hospitals are now being diverted to other purposes, opening up a Pandora's box of questions. Who has the right to sell nonprofit assets, and by what rules? How does the community get compensated in the process? What of the poor and charity care? In short, how do you protect the communities at risk?

When hospital sales skyrocketed during the early 1990s, there were abundant examples of communities getting short-changed in the process. Nearly all the sales were conducted in secret, without community knowledge or input. Some communities got few or no legally binding assurances that the new owner would continue services, provide care to the poor, or even operate their hospital. Troubling reports of private inurement, deliberate misrepresentations, and conflicts of interest were rampant.

Attorneys general, the highest legal authority in the states, turned this situation around. Leaders such as California's Attorney General Dan Lungren saw the need to define rules for such conversions and became advocates for active oversight. As overseers of charitable assets, Lungren and others insisted on a fair and open process, often with public hearings to educate and provide a forum for the community, and they encouraged other attorneys general to do the same. With the backing of the courts and state legislatures, attorneys general contested the worst of the sale deals and, in many states, created an efficient and fair oversight process.

An informed board of directors is essential and integral to the process. Under federal and state laws the boards of not-for-profit hospitals have a fiduciary duty to keep the assets dedicated to their charitable purposes. In deciding to sell a hospital—or redeploy those assets—and in completing the sale process, board members must demonstrate that they are acting in the best interests of the community. They must be unfettered by conflicts of interest or promises of personal gain. They must be sure they are receiving fair market value for the hospital and that the proceeds of the deal are appropriately redirected within the community.

The onus on the board is immense, an onus made all the greater by the dearth of guidance—until now. Here, authors James Schwartz and Chet Horn have created a blueprint for effective board oversight and action. This book provides, for the first time, a clear and articulate description of fiduciary duty as it pertains to hospital conversions. It sets out and defines a process for strategic decision making. It provides guidance on what boards and management must consider and differences among sale structures. It explains the appropriate use of sale proceeds and how to create and direct a foundation or other successor organization. It reviews doctrines of trust law, including *cy pres*. Most important, Schwartz and Horn convey the gravity of fiduciary duty, stressing that with the legal authority to sell hospitals comes enormous responsibility to do it wisely.

No attorney general's office in the country has seen more hospital sales and conversions than California's. And Schwartz and Horn, the deputy attorneys general for charitable trusts, have been on the front line daily, doing the analyses, carrying out the reviews. It is a testament to their skill and experience that all who have dealt with them remark on their fairness, firmness, and vision. They came steeped in charitable-trust law and are now the nation's experts on not-for-profit hospital sales and conversions. Reading this book is truly learning at the knee of the master.

Anyone—board member, community activist, hospital executive, physician, or lawyer—contemplating the sale and conversion of a not-for-profit hospital or other health care institution to a for-profit entity should read this book. It is written with compassion and wisdom; and it is indispensable for not-for-profit boards of directors. Such a guide is long overdue.

Much is at stake in the sale of community not-for-profit hospitals, which have been the backbone of the health care system and the provider of last resort for vulnerable populations. This book is an effort to make sure that when and if nonprofit boards decide to sell community hospitals, they are armed with the information and know-how to meet their highest calling as holders-in-trust of their community-owned, not-for-profit institutions.

Introduction

We recognize that this is a difficult time to be a director or trustee of a nonprofit community hospital or other local, nonprofit health care facility. The conventional wisdom seems to be that community hospitals are dinosaurs whose time on this earth as independent entities is coming to an end and that sooner or later they will all have to enter into strategic alliances—either through mergers into large nonprofit systems or through conversion and strategic partnerships with for-profit chains.

We are not sure that this view is correct. We are sure, however, that in an increasingly competitive health care industry directors and trustees of stand-alone nonprofit hospitals and health care facilities feel under severe pressure. Managed care, industry consolidation, acquisition-minded for-profit hospital chains, increased attention from state attorneys general and the media, and ongoing federal compliance audits have done nothing to ease these pressures. There is some support for the notion that while greed drove the conversions of health-maintenance organizations (HMOs) in the 1980s, fear is driving hospital conversions now.

This book is largely about *conversions*—transactions that result in the transfer of ownership or control of a material amount of the assets of a nonprofit hospital or health facility to the for-profit sector. Whether the specific transaction is an outright sale, a joint venture, or a strategic alliance with physicians, if the end result is that a formerly charitable institution is being operated as a for-profit entity, the transaction is a conversion. And although the proceeds paid to the nonprofit corporation as a result of the conversion continue to be impressed with a trust for charitable purposes, the "converted" operating hospital or health care facility is subject to no such trust. Those institutions have become part of a for-profit operation whose primary goal, quite properly, is to make a profit for its owners. This redeployment of charitable assets defines the conversion process.

This book is, first and foremost, for directors and trustees who voluntarily give their time and their talents to manage their community's nonprofit hospitals and health facilities—an increasingly difficult and underappreciated task. It is our hope that this book will provide them with the tools to guide them through the strategic-planning process and to assist them in dealing with the challenges posed by today's changing health care environment. We also hope that the book is of value to professionals in this area, whether they are hospital or health-facility managers, lawyers, investment bankers, accountants, or consultants. Health-facility directors and trustees rely on these individuals to advise them in the strategic-planning process, and we believe it is helpful, if not essential, for these professionals to understand how state regulators view the complex issues involved in every conversion transaction.

We have tried to provide nonprofit directors and trustees with the advice necessary for meeting their trust responsibilities. If directors understand the legal obligations they accept when they agree to serve on the board of a nonprofit corporation (Chapter One), they will be prepared to meet those obligations. If directors understand the benefits of ongoing strategic planning (Chapter Two), they will be prepared to manage their institution and deal with ever-changing market forces. If directors understand the inherent conflicts of interest facing their senior managers and the consultants advising them in the conversion process (Chapter Two), they will be prepared to critically evaluate the advice being given to the board. If directors understand the fundamental terms of the transactions proposed for their facilities (Chapter Three), they will be prepared to comply with their obligations as charitable trustees. And if directors understand the legal restrictions on the proceeds from a sale or joint-venture transaction (Chapters Four and Five), they will be prepared to create a plan for the use of those proceeds that complies with the law and benefits the community.

The board of directors or trustees is the first and most important line of defense in safeguarding charitable interests once the issue of conversion arises. And we mean the entire board, not just the board chairperson or the management committee. Too often, critical decisions are made by a small group of board members who are not adequately exposed to different points of view. This kind of decision making defeats the purpose of having board members diverse in experience, background, and talent. If all board members have a basic knowledge of their fiduciary obligations and actively participate in the decision-making process (Chapter Six), both they and their institutions will be able to address the challenges of the future. This book is intended to assist in that process.

We feel we are uniquely qualified to provide this assistance. The California attorney general's office has been, we believe, the nation's leader in protecting charitable assets in nonprofit-hospital conversions. From 1995 to 1998, we personally reviewed fifteen separate transactions, involving sixteen acute-care hospitals and additional HMOs, management-service organizations (MSOs), and other ancillary businesses with a total value in excess of $2 billion. We drafted California's hospital conversion law (AB 3101—Isenberg) and the regulations implementing it. We wrote the protocol for reviewing hospital conversions that is being used by several state attorneys general. We provided instruction on how to review conversion transactions for the offices of attorneys general in other states. We created "model-deal" forms that allow the free market to work and that protect charitable assets.

Now for a few disclaimers. The opinions, conclusions, and content of this work do not reflect the official views of the Office of the California Attorney General or any other agency of the State of California. No property, equipment, personnel, or other resources of the State of California have been used in the preparation of this work. Rather, it is the work of and reflects only the views of the authors as individuals.

We have attempted to address the critical issues that are likely to arise in planning for any health care alliance or conversion. However, every specific transaction is different and needs to be analyzed individually by professionals competent to do so. Nonprofit directors and trustees will need the advice of their managers, attorneys, and consultants to properly address a specific proposal. Our goal has been simple. We have tried to provide directors and trustees with sufficient general background to enable them to ask the right questions and critically evaluate the answers they get. If directors use the tools provided in this book, they should feel confident that they can address intelligently and thoroughly any strategic proposal presented to them for approval.

Senior managers, attorneys, accountants, investment bankers, and consultants can give directors and trustees the advice they need to assess the wisdom of specific proposals. But the ultimate responsibility for any strategic decision rests squarely with the directors and trustees. So they need to make sure that their advisers give them the information they need to make that decision carefully, wisely, and with confidence.

1

Fiduciary Obligations

Fiduciary obligations are the rules that directors of nonprofit organizations must obey in their oversight of charitable assets. It does not matter whether your organization is a trust or a nonprofit corporation, you must comply with your fiduciary obligations. If you do not, you breach your trust. Breaches of trust can have serious consequences, including removal from the board, personal liability, and, in the most extreme cases, criminal prosecution. Just as the Hippocratic oath admonishes physicians to "first do no harm," nonprofit-hospital directors are admonished to "first breach no trust."

We discuss trustees' fiduciary duties in the framework of nonprofit-hospital conversions. However, any nonprofit entity can be "converted." These fiduciary duties, therefore, apply equally to directors and trustees of all types of nonprofit corporations—whether they are home health agencies, skilled-nursing facilities, universities, or grant-making foundations. If you are a director or trustee of any charitable corporation, these rules apply to you.

The law imposes three basic duties on nonprofit directors: loyalty, due care, and obedience to purpose. These duties are interrelated. An improper self-dealing arrangement by one director (a breach of the duty of loyalty by that director) may lead to a breach of the duty of due care on the part of other directors who fail to prevent or who ratify the initial breach of trust. We will explain each of these duties and provide common sense advice on how to fulfill them. For those with a greater interest in the subject, we have included in Appendix B a detailed discussion of the legal duties of fiduciaries with reference to appropriate legal authorities. However, the material in this chapter should provide directors and trustees with the basics needed to understand the obligations the law imposes on them as fiduciaries.

Duty of Obedience to Charitable Purpose

Obedience to the charitable purposes of the corporation is the paramount duty of directors. To understand the duty of obedience to purpose, you must recognize that charitable corporations do not own their assets as for-profit corporations do. Rather, charitable corporations and their boards of directors are the trustees of those assets: they hold them "in trust" on behalf of the public for the purposes set forth in the articles of incorporation. Therefore, the directors of a nonprofit corporation have an obligation to manage the charitable assets in a manner that carries out the trust purposes.

In the context of the conversion of nonprofit hospitals, this is a particularly critical issue. Selling your nonprofit hospital to a for-profit corporation represents a fundamental change in the charitable mission of the nonprofit corporation that used to own the hospital. The conversion of a nonprofit hospital spells the end of the hospital's charitable mission. Even though the community may benefit from the hospital's continued operation as a for-profit facility, the hospital itself no longer has a charitable mission. The new owners of the hospital, even in a joint venture in which the charitable corporation is a part owner, will operate the hospital as a for-profit entity.

Step 1: Find Out Whether You Can Convert Your Hospital at All

The charitable corporation that survives the conversion process will have a new mission—to use the proceeds from the sale (and any other assets it keeps) to carry out the charitable purposes of the corporation. Therefore, the first question that nonprofit board members considering a conversion must ask is whether their duty to comply with the corporation's charitable purposes allows them to choose this path at all. You can answer this question by making the following checks:

1. Check your state's charitable-trust law.
2. Check your articles of incorporation, bylaws, and all amendments.
3. Check for restrictions contained in any major gifts, especially large capital-improvement funds.

The first step a nonprofit board considering a conversion must take is to decide what its charitable trust is and then determine whether the proposed transaction is a legally permissible means of carrying out that trust. The laws of the state of incorporation (and of the state where you have your headquarters if it is different), the nonprofit's articles of incorporation and bylaws, and any restrictions imposed by those who have made large donations to your hospital will determine the scope of your trust obligations and whether conversion is possible.

Different states have different rules for conversions of nonprofit corporations. Some general rules may apply. Those states that have adopted the American Bar Association's Revised Model Non-Profit Corporation Act permit the conversion of nonprofit hospitals provided that the conversion proceeds are used for proper charitable purposes. The Model Act specifically authorizes nonprofit corporations to sell all or substantially all of their assets. Without a state law permitting such sales, there is a serious legal question whether a nonprofit community hospital can sell its facility to or enter into a joint venture with a for-profit entity without obtaining court approval under the standards for modifying a charitable trust. These are difficult standards to meet. Generally, a court will require a nonprofit to prove that it is impossible or impractical to continue operating the hospital without facing financial ruin. So your first order of business in considering a conversion proposal is to have your corporation's counsel advise you about the options allowed under the laws of your state.

Second, you must decide whether the charitable trust described in your corporation's articles of incorporation or bylaws effectively prevents the conversion. For example, in a California case, a hospital's articles of incorporation limited the use of its assets to the operation of a nonprofit community hospital in a specific city. No other charitable uses of the assets were allowed. Therefore, if the hospital were to be sold, all the proceeds of the sale and other assets of the corporation would have to have been transferred to another nonprofit hospital operating in that city. That option was not acceptable to either the nonprofit seller or the for-profit buyer, and as a result the deal was called off.

Third, gift restrictions in your original endowment may also limit your options. If initial gifts used to build or acquire your nonprofit hospital contained a requirement that the hospital always be operated as a nonprofit facility, that requirement must be obeyed, and you will not be allowed to enter into a conversion transaction.

Before you even begin considering a conversion transaction, have your attorneys complete each of the three checks of Step 1. The duty of obedience to purpose is the first issue that you and your lawyers must address. If you do not, you may be personally liable for charitable funds wasted on pursuing a legally impermissible venture. By way of analogy, would you retain and pay a general contractor to build a real estate project before determining whether the zoning laws permitted the project?

Step 2: Determine How You Can Spend the Charity's Money

You can use the following three criteria to decide whether your plan for spending the charity's money complies with the duty of obedience to purpose:

1. Determine the charitable trust that governs your assets.

2. Find out how you can spend your money legally.

3. Develop plans for spending that follow the advice of your attorneys or duplicate or closely resemble your hospital's historical expenditures.

Even if a transaction is permissible and the assets retained by the surviving charity can be used to fund a grant-making foundation, that foundation's discretion to use the fund may be severely limited. Your board will be frustrated if it sells the hospital with the expectation that the proceeds can be used for specific purposes (such as homeless shelters or education scholarships) only to discover that the law limits expenditure of the sale proceeds solely to hospital and related medical purposes. In fact, sometimes this limitation will negate the purpose for which the board sold the hospital, and it will be left with neither a hospital nor the ability to pursue the alternative charitable programs it had planned. This, too, is a threshold issue that you should address before you decide to sell the hospital.

So what can a board do if it decides that conversion is the right solution for its community, but its attorneys advise that charitable-trust problems may prohibit that option? If economic conditions justify a proposed conversion, the local court has the power to authorize conversion upon a proper showing. But be careful: asking the court to approve a conversion has risks. If the court determines that a nonprofit board is attempting to sell its hospital without adequate justification, the court can remove the board members who approved the attempt and appoint different trustees to take over operation of the hospital (for a description of a case where this risk arose, see the discussion of *Estate of Beryl Buck* in Appendix B).

The best advice we can offer:

- Retain legal counsel knowledgeable in charitable-trust law.

- Have your attorneys advise you of the permitted uses of the charitable assets.

- Read your articles of incorporation, bylaws, and key gift documents. Often they are written in reasonably plain

English and will alert you to potential limits on how
you can spend the charity's money.

- Treat the future spending plan as a threshold issue. Do
  not go down the conversion path until you are sure
  that the law allows you to spend the conversion proceeds in ways that are acceptable to your board.

Duty of Loyalty

The duty of loyalty is another key obligation imposed on directors
of charitable corporations. Simply put, this duty precludes directors from taking unfair advantage of their position to enrich themselves or members of their families at the expense of the charitable
corporation. Commonly referred to as "self-dealing" or as "related-
party transactions," violations of this rule create the greatest risk of
personal liability on the part of directors for two reasons. First, enforcement agencies give violations of this duty the highest priority.
Second, directors' and officers' liability insurance and the business
judgment rule (as explained later in this chapter) do not offer protection for self-dealing transactions.

In most states, self-dealing transactions are not automatically illegal, and some types of self-dealing transactions are specifically
allowed according to prescribed rules. It is important to distinguish
legally permissible self-dealing from that which can result in removal from the board or worse.

The most valuable advice we can give you is to understand that
rules differ from state to state and to learn how they apply in your
state. For example, prior to the enactment of the new Nonprofit
Corporation Law in 1980, the U.S. District Court for the Northern
District of California (interpreting California law) prohibited all
self-dealing. This strict trust law interpretation contrasted with the
decision of the U.S. District Court for the District of Columbia,
which had, two years earlier, rejected that standard in favor of a

more permissive corporate standard that allows some self-dealing if it is in the corporation's interest. Thus, a transaction that would be legal within the District of Columbia could, in California, create a potential for personal liability.

The law does not treat all types of self-dealing the same way. Under current law in California, for example, some self-dealing transactions are permissible. However, loans to directors are never legal unless approved in advance and in writing by the state attorney general.

Therefore, if you are considering a transaction that may involve self-dealing with one of your board members, insist that the board take each of the following actions:

- Disclose *all* facts about the transaction to the *entire* board.

- Obtain a written opinion from your attorney advising the board about the rules that govern self-dealing in your state.

- Require your attorney to provide an unconditional opinion letter assuring that the transaction does not violate the rules.

Without that opinion, no director can be sure that he or she is complying with the law. Be sure to document the professional advice given to you, as well as every step taken by the board in approving a self-dealing transaction. Virtually every state that permits self-dealing requires that a number of specific findings be made by the board before it approves a self-dealing transaction. Failure to jump through these hoops can make improper a transaction that might otherwise have been allowed.

In nonprofit-hospital conversions, breaches of the duty of loyalty generally happen in one of two ways. Board members either (1) engage in classic self-dealing with the charitable corporation or (2) use their position to obtain monetary benefits from the acquiring for-profit entity, a practice known as profiteering. Examples of both these situations are much too easy to find. To give an obvious example, self-dealing occurs when directors vote to authorize payments to themselves from the proceeds of the sale of the hospital. These payments can be "golden parachutes," enhanced retirement benefits, agreements not to compete, and so on. These types of payments are always suspect and often illegal. At worst, they constitute a fraudulent distribution of charitable funds, which can be a criminal offense.

Profiteering by directors is usually more subtle (and more difficult to discover), but no less improper. It occurs, for example, if a director causes the for-profit buyer to purchase property or business interests owned by the director at an inflated price or to overpay for joint business ventures in which the director and the hospital are partners. If you let such profiteering happen, you face personal liability for the results.

Conversions are complex legal transactions, and the duty of loyalty is sometimes difficult to interpret. However, following a few simple rules will guide you in making the right decisions:

- Act with the highest degree of good faith as a fiduciary.

- Avoid conflicts of interest and self-dealing.

- If self-dealing is legal in your state

    Make sure the transaction is principally for the benefit of the charity and not the involved director.

    Fully disclose the interest of the involved director to the board.

    Make sure the charity could not have obtained a better deal from someone else.

In your effort to follow these rules, especially those concerning self-dealing, ask yourself and other board members the following questions. Would the board have entered into the transaction if it did not involve a director? If the answer is no, you probably do not want to vote to approve the deal. Do you understand all the reasons why the proposed self-dealing transaction is good for the corporation? If not, you and the other board members probably do not know all the facts, and suspicion will exist with regard to any subsequent ratification by the board. Does the transaction meet the "best deal in town" test? If not, or if you do not know, then the transaction should be avoided. As a practical matter, the best way to ensure that a self-dealing transaction satisfies the law is to insist that written bids be secured from alternative sources for the services in question or, in sales of charitable assets, to obtain proof that all potential buyers were contacted and that the best price possible was obtained.

If you get the appropriate answers to each of these questions and document your steps to comply with local laws about self-dealing, you will at least have met the standards of the American Bar Association's Model Act. If you cannot meet these tests and prove that you have met them, your level of personal exposure is probably too high.

Duty of Due Care

The duty of due care refers to the directors' obligation to exercise diligence in making decisions involving charitable assets. Because most director decisions involve this duty, it is extremely important to understand the legal requirements imposed by it. As in the case of the duty of loyalty, the specific level of diligence to which directors are held varies from state to state.

States have generally applied one of two standards to directors of nonprofit corporations—the corporate-law standard or a quasi-trust-law standard. At the risk of oversimplifying the rules, the corporate-law standard generally provides that if directors make an adequate inquiry before reaching or approving a decision, that decision cannot be challenged if the directors' belief that the decision was in the corporation's interest has a rational basis. This is not a difficult standard to meet. The quasi-trust-law standard, however, imposes liability on directors if their decision does not meet the standard of care that an "ordinarily prudent person" would use. This standard is more stringent than the corporate standard and always poses the risk that a court, looking at a transaction years after the fact, will disagree with the decision made by a nonprofit board.

Fortunately for directors, the duty of due care, regardless of the standard of care imposed, can be satisfied by creating and following the proper decision-making process. Your attorneys can—and you should insist that they do—create a process for your board's decisions that will protect members from exposure to personal liability.

Despite the ease with which the duty of due care can be satisfied, it is frequently violated. These violations can result in embarrassing breach-of-trust lawsuits against directors who acted without any ill motive and who did not profit from their actions. The question routinely asked by such directors is, How can this be? The answer is that the directors or their counsel failed to create a proper decision-making process.

The key point is that virtually all breach-of-trust actions against directors for violating the duty of due care are preventable if these steps are taken:

- Delegate responsibility for decisions to qualified board committees or experts.

- Document and rely on the advice given to you by those to whom you delegated the responsibility.

- Take advantage of the business judgment rule by making a reasonable inquiry before you make a final decision.

The law in virtually all states allows nonprofit directors to *delegate responsibility* for decisions to committees of the board of directors, to corporate officers, or to outside experts and consultants. Even in states like California, which impose the quasi-trust-law standard of care, directors are allowed to delegate this responsibility. It is, therefore, never an excuse to say, "I didn't have time to look into this matter or to investigate it fully." This is not an excuse; it is an admission of liability.

Not surprisingly, the law permits board members to *rely on the advice* received from those to whom they have delegated responsibility for particular decisions. For example, if you have retained an investment banker to advise you as to the value of the nonprofit hospital, you are permitted to rely on his or her advice. Doing so will, in almost all cases, immunize you from potential liability. However, you should carefully *document the advice* you get and the process the board followed in considering that advice.

Finally, you should be aware that *the business judgment rule is applicable* to decisions made pursuant to the duty of due care. The business judgment rule is a court-created doctrine that protects directors from liability for business decisions that turn out badly if those directors conducted a reasonable inquiry prior to making the decision. Always take these steps, which are the minimum necessary to ensure that your decision-making process is sufficient to invoke the protection of this rule:

- Act in good faith while making your decision.

- Consider all relevant facts and ignore none.

- Demonstrate and document that your reliance was reasonable.

- Do not engage in self-dealing. (The business judgment rule does not apply to self-dealing in most states.)

If you want to rely on the advice of the investment banker mentioned above under the duty of due care, do not hire your brother-in-law to provide the advice; do not sell to a company in which you hold a material financial interest; read the materials submitted to you before you vote; and do not have the hospital take back a note from the purchaser after being advised by a fellow board member of a *Wall Street Journal* article that reports that the acquiring company is considering filing for bankruptcy protection.

Conclusion

Complying with these three duties—obedience to purpose, loyalty, and due care—is not brain surgery, and it is not difficult to do properly. Create a process that places responsibility for doing due diligence on those persons with the background, skill, and time to do it properly. Make sure those individuals provide written recommendations to the board. Discuss those recommendations at a board meeting and determine whether anyone is aware of contrary information. Document your decision in board minutes and explain the rationale for that decision. Good faith and a proper process can and will ensure that you comply with your duties.

2

Strategic Planning

In this chapter, we will provide you with steps to successful strategic planning for health-facility conversions and strategic alliances. These steps are neither complicated nor arcane, but they will greatly improve your chances of reaching a result that meets your goals while retaining the trust and respect of your community. Without proper strategic planning, hospital conversions and alliances can exemplify the worst in crisis management, and the result is often conflict with the community, internal board friction, hastily devised and ineffective strategies, wasted money, and, in the worst case, illegal or imprudent acts that expose board members to personal liability. So follow the steps, do it right, and you and your community will be better off for the effort.

Proper strategic planning is at the heart of every successful decision. It provides decision makers with the tools to identify their available options, carefully evaluate those options, and then make a reasoned decision as to how best to serve their institution and their community. Too often, particularly in hospital conversions, the decision-making process has been severely compromised by improper planning or failure to plan. In our experience, senior management invariably does the initial planning leading to strategic alliances. All too often, the board, or at least most board members, are kept in the dark until a transaction has been all but completed. The rationale for this process is usually a need for secrecy to prevent the financial damage to the institution that might arise from disclosing that the hospital is "in play." Although this is a legitimate concern, it cannot justify board members' violating their fiduciary duties, especially the duty of due care, which requires every board member to make an informed and reasoned decision.

We have seen cases where management cloaked its strategic planning in secrecy to prevent the full board from adequately exploring all available options. Then, under the pressure of a perceived fiscal or management crisis, the board was asked to approve a proposed transaction without ever having had the opportunity to explore alternative options or, worse, to fully understand the terms of the specific transaction being submitted to them for a vote. The simple fact is that such crises rarely happen overnight. And further, this management style negates the advantage of having a board diverse in experience, talent, and outlook. The decision to convert a hospital to for-profit status and change the nature of the institution so that it becomes a grant-making foundation is the single most important decision each board member will ever consider. This judgment requires the highest—not the lowest—level of discussion and is never properly delegated solely to senior management.

Five steps are necessary to ensure that strategic planning is done properly:

1. Get the entire board involved early and take control of the decision-making process.

2. Identify legally permissible options.

3. Assemble the right team of management and experts to identify the problems and recommend solutions.

4. Create a decision-making process that lets you shape your options to meet your goals and works with your community, not against it.

5. Allow enough time to make an informed and reasoned decision.

Step 1: Get the Board Involved Early

The first issue a board should address is, What are our real options and where do they lead us? The earlier the board begins the process of identifying its options, the more options it is likely to have because it will have more time to discover them. Time is the most precious commodity in dealing with changing circumstances. If you as board members are kept apprised of financial developments and see adverse trends developing, you can ask your management to provide you with a full range of possible solutions. These solutions can cover a broad range:

- Revise the business plan to meet market conditions.

- Develop strategic partnerships with local providers such as physician groups and clinics.

- Enter into joint operating agreements or other affiliations with other local hospitals.

- Affiliate with a large nonprofit system.

- Sell your facility to or enter into a joint venture or other strategic partnership with a for-profit hospital company.

With adequate time and by following the right steps, you will be able to explore each of these options and make the decision that you feel is best for your hospital and your community. In every case we have reviewed, when lack of timely board involvement stripped the board of its options, the results were poor decision making, which exposed the board to criticism from its community, and sometimes liability for inadvertently breaching the trust on which the board held its assets.

Thus, the most important key to successful strategic planning decisions is control of the decision-making process by the board from the very beginning. You should require your hospital's chief executive officer (or whoever will lead the planning process) to advise the board whenever serious consideration is being given to a merger, sale, joint venture, or other transaction of major concern to the hospital. Once the process of consideration has begun, require the planners to keep the board apprised of developments on an ongoing and regular basis.

The beginning of the planning process is the time to instruct your management to bring all options to the attention of the board so that the board can meet its fiduciary obligations in making the ultimate decision. If you leave the planning process solely to your chief executive officer or chief operating officer, you will be limited to the choices that officer brings you. Senior managers worried about their personal futures may well have goals or priorities for the conversion decision that are different from the board's and from the goals that will best serve the interests of the community. The ultimate responsibility for any decision rests on the board's shoulders; the board should control the process leading to that decision.

Step 2: Identify the Legally Permissible Options

Once the board has taken control of the strategic-planning process, the next step is to identify the universe of legally permissible options.

Determine Restrictions

If conversion to for-profit is one option that is being considered, there are two sources of possible limitations on the conversion choices available to your charity.

- Your state's charitable-trust law either may prevent you from considering a conversion at all or may limit the conversion formats you can consider.

- Your own corporate documents, including your articles of incorporation and any major gift instruments restricting your use of donations, can affect the choices available to you.

Different states impose different statutory restrictions on the form that conversions, if permitted at all, can take. New York law, for example, effectively prohibits sales of nonprofit hospitals to publicly traded companies. Michigan law may preclude joint ventures between nonprofit hospitals and for-profit corporations completely. A California statute effectively prohibits any insider purchases of nonprofit hospitals, and an IRS Revenue Ruling may prohibit virtually all currently used forms of joint ventures. So the first thing you need to do when planning for a possible conversion is to have your attorneys identify any statutory or common law limitations on the available options in your state.

As we noted in Chapter One, the scope of a nonprofit corporation's charitable trust is usually defined by its articles of incorporation. Nonprofit hospitals have a wide range of charitable-purpose clauses in their articles of incorporation. We have seen articles with clauses as sweeping as permitting any activity that supports charitable, educational, or scientific purposes and as narrow as requiring the perpetual operation of a nonprofit hospital in a specific city. It should be obvious that the hospital with sweeping corporate purposes is going to have greater flexibility in choosing future strategic plans than the hospital with a narrow corporate purpose. What may not be obvious is that a narrow charitable-purpose clause may effectively prevent any conversion of the hospital.

Avoid Common Errors

Review of corporate articles is, therefore, the starting point for a strategic-planning process. We need, however, to warn you of four common errors boards make when reviewing corporate articles:

- Reviewing the wrong articles of incorporation
- Reviewing only the articles of incorporation
- Ignoring the hospital's operating history
- Trying to change the trust terms by amending the articles of incorporation

Boards sometimes *review the wrong articles of incorporation* because many nonprofit hospitals and hospital systems have both a parent corporation (which may have extremely broad corporate purposes) and separate independent hospital corporations (which actually hold all the hospital assets being sold and which have narrower purposes). In planning for a sale, joint venture, or other strategic partnership, the articles of incorporation of the independent hospitals define the trust on which the assets are held, not those of the parent corporation.

Also, the most recent revision of the corporation's articles may not define the trust on which the assets are held. Corporations can and often do revise their articles, including the statement of corporate purpose. The allowable corporate purposes—and the trust on which the assets are held—may have changed over time. This change creates differing rules for different assets, depending on when they were obtained. Generally, the trust restrictions that apply to a specific asset are those that were in effect at the time the asset was acquired.

Tip! To properly conduct a strategic-planning analysis in this area, the board needs to review all the articles of the corporation from its inception to the date of the review. Only then will the board be able to identify the possible limitations that might be imposed by the regulatory authority that will review a proposed affiliation.

Review of the articles of incorporation alone will not give enough information to properly define your charity's trust obligations. Hospitals often have accepted restricted gifts that govern some or all of their assets. The original founders of the hospital may, by restrictions in gift documents, have created specific limitations on how the assets of the hospital can be used. Those limitations may have important implications for the ability of the corporation to change the nature of the corporate charitable purposes.

Tip! A board considering affiliation possibilities must conduct a thorough review of all significant gift documents, especially those related to the initial founding of the hospital or to large gifts, because they may contain restrictions on use that limit the nonprofit's options.

The final component of your charity's trust definition will be found in *the operating history of your hospital.* Therefore, it is most important that the board understand the operational history of its facility. Courts look to the historical operations of charities to help define the nature of the charitable trust that they are bound by. Even if you have a broad statement of purposes in your articles, if you have always operated as a hospital, that operating history will likely define the nature of your charitable trust. The courts are likely to define your predominant charitable purpose as operating a hospital and restrict your post-conversion use of the proceeds to similar purposes. The board must realize that if the scope of the charitable trust governing your facility is limited to the operation or support of a nonprofit hospital, that restriction will significantly limit how the proceeds of a conversion transaction can be spent.

Directors will often attempt to get around some of these charitable-trust problems by simply *amending the articles of incorporation.* But changing the trust in this way does not work. Any amendment of your articles can affect only subsequently obtained assets; all "old" assets are still governed by the specific articles of incorporation that were in effect when they were obtained.

Tip! If the use of the proceeds following a sale or other type of conversion is critical to your decision to go forward, the time to make sure you can accomplish what you want is before you undertake the enormous expense of going through the conversion process. If you want to have a general, health care grant-making foundation at the end of the process, then be sure that such a foundation is allowed under your state law and governing instruments. If it is not, you do not want to spend hundreds of thousands of dollars going through a process that will end in futility.

In sum, not every option will be available to every institution. Your choices will depend on what is permissible under your state's charitable-trust law in light of the corporate documents governing your institution and its operational history. Finding out what options are open to your institution simply cannot be avoided or deferred if the board anticipates spending significant sums of money to engage in planning for a possible conversion. Make no mistake, a thorough planning process leading to the development of strategic options for your hospital will be expensive. No amount of planning will permit a nonprofit board to enter into strategic arrangements that are prohibited by its corporate charter or governing law. If you spend large amounts of money seeking approval for such arrangements, you expose yourself to the risk of personal liability for all such expenditures.

Step 3: Assemble the Right Team of Experts to Work with Your Management, Identify the Problems, and Recommend Solutions

Few nonprofit hospital boards possess the expertise to understand fully the complex market forces affecting their hospital and the appropriate responses to them. Accordingly, the board's duty is to design a process for securing advice from persons or firms that do have that expertise. The board will, quite naturally, look to hospital management for the first level of advice on what is happening in the hospital's market. Hospital management usually consist of both experienced business managers and medical practitioners. They can, and typically do, provide the board with ongoing reports of the hospital's financial condition and the forces affecting that condition. Hospital managers can also be expected to be familiar with the larger forces of change in the delivery of health care that may have an impact on the hospital's future. If your hospital has specific financial problems, management will be the best source for information about the problems and their impact on the hospital.

However, hospital management may not be in the best position to provide unbiased advice concerning solutions. Indeed, the board must always keep in mind the natural conflict of interest hospital managers have—protecting their own jobs. Even a cursory review of conversion transactions shows that senior managers of the affected hospitals can receive lucrative employment offers from the acquiring entity. In the end the board must be able to satisfy itself that the possibility of increased compensation did not influence the advice management provided to the board or the board's decision.

In addition to relying on management for advice, the board should retain independent outside experts to provide advice about market conditions affecting the hospital and possible solutions, from simple cost-containment strategies to outright sale. The key to a successful process is that the experts retained by the board be independent from management. If the experts serve merely as surrogates for management, the board will not have eliminated the problems inherent in relying solely on senior management. These problems include both a natural reluctance to provide the board with financial information that reflects poorly on management as well as conflicts posed by management's potential for receiving lucrative personal financial packages from a for-profit acquirer.

To address this conflict of interest on the part of management, the California legislature enacted a statute restricting the ability of boards to rely on senior managers in for-profit conversions if the managers intend to seek employment or other compensation from the buyer (S.B. 413, effective October 1, 1997). The statute prohibits boards from "substantially relying" on the advice of senior managers who have not signed a declaration that they do not intend to seek employment with the purchasing entity. If managers are not willing to sign such declarations, the board may rely on their advice concerning a proposed transaction only if it has engaged independent experts to review that information and advice. The statute also prohibits members of the board who negotiate the terms of the sale from receiving, directly or indirectly, any compensation, payment, or other form of remuneration from the purchaser, except for health care professionals who provide patient care after the sale. If your state lacks such a law, you might wish to adopt it for your charity by adding it to your bylaws.

Once the board has selected its advisory team, the first task of the advisers will be to describe accurately the current market conditions affecting the hospital and to project, within the limits of forecasting capability, the impact such conditions will have on the hospital's future. When the board is armed with that information, the experts can identify the range of options for addressing whatever problems the hospital faces. For example, if a hospital is facing declining revenues because of lower payments from insurers and declining bed occupancy, it may be possible to solve those problems without a conversion by trimming services, cutting costs, or rationalizing facility use with nearby hospitals or clinics. If those approaches will not fix the problems, steps such as partnering, affiliating with other nonprofit institutions, or conversion can be considered. The key point is that the board's decision-making process needs to be informed by an accurate understanding of the problems that need to be addressed.

Tip! Use the business expertise of your senior managers in considering conversion options, but remember their potential conflicts. The best way to guard against bad advice by managers is to ensure that independent experts provide advice to the board unfiltered by possible management bias.

Step 4: Shape Your Options to Meet Your Goals and Work with Your Community

Once your advisers have given you their best forecast for the hospital's future, they will be in a position to suggest the range of choices the board has. Before they can do that, however, the advisers will have to understand clearly the board's goals, the criteria the board will use to choose the ultimate option, and the needs of the community that the board wants to have met at the end of the conversion process.

Meeting Your Goals

The board must set up a decision-making process that clearly establishes and communicates the board's goals to the team of advisers it has assembled. That decision-making process should also clearly set out the criteria that the board will use in selecting among the available options. Unless the board sets out the goals and the criteria it will use, it risks losing control of the ultimate decision. That loss of control could result in the waste of large amounts of money in pursuit of choices the board would never consider. For example, a board does itself no favor if it allows its advisory team to evaluate for-profit alternatives if the board is not willing to consider them. Similarly, if your state law prohibits joint ventures with for-profit companies, you waste any money spent evaluating that option.

Assuming that your state law and governing trust documents allow you broad discretion over the shape of your charity's future, you should develop the criteria you want to use to evaluate your advisers' suggested options. The process for developing such criteria can be as formal or informal as you wish. However, our experience shows that including the broadest array of affected constituencies—by informing and soliciting the views of employees, doctors, management, and the community—will help smooth the conversion process.

The affiliation criteria your board selects will be greatly influenced by whether it is limiting itself to nonprofit or for-profit partners. If you are considering only nonprofit partners (for a sale or joint venture), commitment to the hospital mission may not be of much concern, while financial strength or governance issues may be paramount, particularly if you are considering affiliation with a longtime neighbor. Alternatively, if you are considering a for-profit partner, commitment to the hospital's mission statement may be an important concern of your board.

When assessing the importance of any particular criterion, the board should keep in mind a simple but important fact: all conditions imposed on a buyer or partner will have a cost. So you must weigh the perceived need for any particular condition against the likely cost to the charity before you insist on imposing the condition as part of a proposed transaction. An illustration will help make the point. Suppose your board wants to insist that any affiliation with a for-profit company (whether through a sale, joint venture, or other arrangement) will maintain the hospital's historical level of charity care, which has been 4 percent of gross revenue. That company will immediately calculate the impact that condition will have on the future revenue stream from operations, calculate the present value of that impact, and reduce the price they are willing to pay for the hospital accordingly.

Although it may not be as obvious, other conditions will have similar impacts. A board considering whether to impose conditions on prospective affiliation partners needs to have some idea of the cost of those conditions in order to understand their implications and to arrive at an informed decision before imposing them. Determining these costs is an essential part of reasoned decision making and must be undertaken to comply with the duty of due care.

Tip! Make sure that the goals you establish for selling to or engaging in a joint venture with a for-profit company and the criteria you use to make any conversion decision are shaped by the needs of your community as well as by the charitable-trust limits of your institution.

Engaging the Community

Our experience suggests strongly that the conversion process works best if the board works with the community that the hospital has served historically rather than against it. The board's decision-making process should not only seek community input but also include se-lection criteria that demonstrate the board's continuing commit-ment to meet community needs.

Many issues are common to conversion transactions in which the local communities have a stake, including commitment to the hos-pital mission statement, governance after the affiliation, charity-care commitment, regional commitment, maintenance of particular ser-vices at the hospital, physician integration, financial strength, em-ployee commitment, capitalization of system, and economies of scale. A host of variables will determine which of these criteria are important for any particular transaction. We discuss some of the more common criteria here.

We frequently see boards that are either selling their hospital or considering a joint venture with a for-profit company insist that the buyer or potential partner agree to adopt the *hospital's mission state-ment* after the close of the transaction. In sale transactions, this con-dition is often expressed in the form of a contractual right that the seller may enforce by a suit for injunctive relief or damages. In joint ventures, this condition usually is included in the joint-venture op-erating agreement as one of the matters over which the nonprofit members of the joint-venture board will retain veto power. Non-profit board members typically insist on such provisions out of a strongly felt desire to protect the community from a reduction in medical services. However, although such sentiments are laudable and appropriate for boards, boards must have some basis for deter-mining both the enforceability of such terms and their value. In-cluding such criteria in your deal may have price effects, and failure to carefully consider these factors will leave the board open to criticism.

Governance issues rarely arise in the sale context. Few firms will pay tens of millions of dollars for a facility they cannot control on their terms. However, governance issues are crucial in joint ven-tures. They can also arise in leasing arrangements and nonprofit af-filiations. In joint ventures, governance of the joint-venture entity is the key to power sharing in the partnership and is crucial to protecting the nonprofit's equity interest and profit potential. We discuss these issues thoroughly in Chapter Five. In transactions that involve affiliations short of a joint venture (such as leasing, joint buying arrangements, or network affiliations) resolution of governance issues is essential, as they dictate who makes the key decisions. For example, if you join a pooling arrangement with several other hospitals in your service area for the purpose of combining your patient strength to negotiate more favorable terms from insurers, important issues will include who decides how to conduct the negotiations and how payments made by the insurers will be allocated among the pool members. It goes without saying that such important matters require careful attention by the board considering them.

Your board may want to assure that the acquiring firm maintains certain levels of *health care delivery to the community*. Whether you are considering a sale, joint venture, or other conversion format, a variety of contractual provisions can be used to attempt to garner guarantees about continued levels of health care delivery. You should think about the cost of such guarantees and consider alternative methods of achieving the same goals. If you have reviewed the issues, considered relevant information, and consulted with appropriate experts, you will insulate yourselves from later criticism for any decision you make.

Nonprofit hospitals are proud, and rightly so, of their record of providing *care to those who cannot afford to pay for medical services*. Boards may appropriately insist that a for-profit entity acquiring the hospital maintain particular levels of charity care for the community. However, in considering whether to attempt to negotiate such a contractual condition and suffer the downward price adjustment that will accompany it, the board needs to be sure it understands these issues. For example, in most states, acute-care licenses require that hospitals provide emergency treatment without regard to the ability to pay. Accordingly, any charity-care commitment by a for-profit buyer will have to either count such care or not. If that care is going to count toward the charity-care commitment of the contract, then no price adjustments would be appropriate because the buyer would be obligated to provide that type of care in any event. If emergency care is not going to be counted toward the contractual commitment to provide charity care, the nonprofit board needs to think carefully about what kind of programs will count, how much they will cost, who will monitor and enforce the commitment, and many other issues that go along with attempts to impose postclosing obligations on the buyer.

Enforcement issues must also be thought through before insisting on a charity-care commitment because describing the commitment the buyer is assuming is not easy. Do you count contractual discounts from payers, emergency room treatment that goes unpaid, employee education that the hospital sponsors, or community education sponsored by the hospital? Once you define the commitment, how do you monitor whether the buyer is carrying it out? Is it worth your while to insist on the right to review books and records after the close? What happens if the buyer fails to keep its commitment? Will you pay for the cost of litigation to enforce these provisions or rely simply on moral suasion or public pressure? The board needs to carefully consider all these issues and balance them against the benefits to be achieved and alternative methods of securing the same benefits for the community. It is, after all, unwise to discount the price for which you sell your hospital to obtain benefits that your community may never see.

Another issue that arises frequently in the sale of community hospitals is whether the buyer is willing to commit to *maintaining hospital operations in the region* where it is located. We have seen this issue arise after the fact when a purchasing firm buys several hospitals serving a region and then closes one or more of those hospitals. We have also seen this issue arise in the bidding for a single hospital. One example occurred in Southern California when two firms were vying to buy one of the two hospitals serving a fast-growing, but relatively remote, region of the state. One of the competitors was a large for-profit hospital chain seeking to enter that market. The other bidder was the owner of the other local hospital serving that community. Not surprisingly, the local firm was willing to pay more for the privilege of creating a monopoly in that region. In fact, it announced its intention, if it were the winning bidder, to shut the hospital down. The new entrant, however, was willing to commit to expanding the hospital's operations to prepare for anticipated growth in the region. The board of the seller was faced with the choice of accepting the lower offer and ensuring a continued presence for its hospital in the region or accepting the higher price, thereby receiving more funds for its parent nonprofit corporation but suffering the closure of its hospital.

In situations where commitment to the region is a criterion the selling board wants to consider, it must be prepared to face difficult choices. In order to make those choices, the board needs to clarify its goals early in the process and develop a full understanding of all costs that might be associated with the criteria it has chosen to apply to the sale.

If your hospital provides *special services* that are unique in your area, such as a burn unit, a trauma center, or a neonatal unit, you may want to ensure the continued availability of those services to your community. Such specialized services are often money-losing propositions that may not be maintained by the company buying your hospital. If your board thinks that maintaining such services is vital to the community, it can insist that the buyer agree to keep them at the hospital either perpetually (to the extent enforceable) or for a period of years.

Keep in mind that any restrictions you place on the buyer's use of the facility will almost certainly have adverse price effects. So you should evaluate carefully whether requiring the buyer to provide such services is the most cost-effective means of ensuring their availability. For example, it might be more efficient for your charity to contract with some other firm to provide a specialized service to the community as part of its ongoing charitable mission. To know whether that solution is more efficient requires the board to analyze the cost of providing the service over the requisite time period and the price impact of insisting that the buyer provide the service. Absent that analysis, you have no factual basis for deciding between the two options.

Hospital boards often have close ties with their physicians. These ties are born of long affiliations and close working relationships. It is, therefore, not unusual for hospital boards to attempt to build *protections for physicians* into the sale process. An important element of physician concern with any sale is the assurance that the new owner will continue relationships with physician groups that serve the hospital on terms that are favorable to the doctors. Although this concern is understandable, in our view it is not properly a concern for the nonprofit board. The board's fiduciary duties are owed to the charitable beneficiaries of the hospital, not to its physicians or managers. Thus, the board is not free to negotiate special protections for doctors (or any other private group) that will diminish the value received for the charitable assets being sold.

This is not to say that the board may not appropriately consider the views of doctors, nurses, and other groups. These groups are critical to the hospital's continued viability as an important community institution, and that long-term viability is a matter that the board may appropriately factor into its criteria for selecting an affiliation format and partner. The process of developing selection criteria can certainly include mechanisms to solicit the views of physicians, the community, and other affected constituencies. These groups can play an important role in evaluating qualitative issues concerning prospective partners, but the board must always keep in mind that its paramount obligation is to the charitable beneficiaries of the hospital.

The process of deciding which of these issues need to be addressed in a conversion should include securing the views of all affected constituencies. These include the hospital's management, doctors' groups, nurses, employees, and, most important, the community itself. Hospital trustees tend to think of the hospital as "their" hospital, as they are the people charged with the duty to oversee the hospital's operations, protect its assets, and carry out its charitable mission, and they are also the people on the hook for any violation of those duties. They face the risk of potential liability for mistakes and no one else does. Yet trustees need to remember that they are trustees, not owners. They hold the assets in trust for the real owners: the pubic beneficiaries of the institution. Just as for-profit corporations must convince their shareholders that a significant change in corporate direction is in their interest, nonprofit trustees should not overlook the importance of convincing the public that a proposed conversion is in the community's interest.

Failure to get community support for a proposed conversion may well engender confusion, fear, animosity, and opposition, which will make the conversion difficult, if not impossible. Securing the public's support for a proposed conversion from the outset will have the opposite effect. So, as you design your process for considering a possible conversion, consider whether you want to encourage the public to support your efforts or whether you prefer a nasty fight (oftentimes fought on the front pages of your local newspaper) over this important community decision. In our experience, the boards that have taken the time to garner public support for their plans at the earliest stages of the conversion process have experienced the greatest success and the least resistance to the critical decision to sell the community's hospital.

Designing a community-outreach program as part of your conversion process will require careful attention to the unique aspects of your community. An example of outreach efforts that succeeded may point to some useful approaches. In a transaction with a for-profit company in 1996, a Southern California nonprofit hospital hired a consulting firm to convey to the community information that had been developed by the hospital as part of its state-mandated community-needs assessment (a biannual requirement in

California). The needs assessment included interviewing 250 people from the community served by the hospital. Those interviewed included the superintendent of schools, the chief of police, the county sheriff, representatives of the Hispanic Chamber of Commerce, the director of the county public health services department, school principals, the president of the local community college, doctors, business executives, and community members. In addition the senior managers of the hospital personally conducted a door-to-door survey of residents in five areas within two miles of the hospital. The survey sought information concerning the experience of local residents in gaining access to health care at the hospital. Questions that were asked included: What do you feel are the top health issues facing our community? What do you think are some of the barriers to receiving health care in our community? What are some of the ways that we as a community can improve the health status of our community? The hospital participated in a number of focus-group discussions with particular users of the health services provided in the county. These groups consisted of patients and health providers. The hospital used the sessions to test its ideas about community needs as they coalesced from the needs assessments and survey work that was being done. The hospital also reviewed the community-needs assessments done by other nearby hospitals. This information was updated from public sources by the hospital's consultants.

From all the data, the hospital determined the ability of various groups in the community to secure adequate health care. They also determined the areas where improvement in health care delivery was needed and identified at-risk segments of the community for whom adequate health care was virtually nonexistent. Finally, the hospital developed a series of proposals that identified both the means and the agencies that could help address the critical health needs of the community.

With this detailed information, the hospital was well prepared to address issues that might be raised concerning the impact of the proposed conversion on the delivery of health care to its community. This process enabled the nonprofit board to assure the community that the proposed conversion would improve rather than harm health care delivery. These assurances, in turn, allowed the board to garner community support for the transaction. Finally, this process armed the board with information for developing the trust language that would govern the charity's future activities and convincing the California attorney general and the courts that the board's plan satisfied the requirements of trust law.

Step 5: Give Yourself Enough Time to Make a Reasoned Decision

At the outset of this chapter, we advised you to make sure that the board takes control of the conversion planning process from the earliest stages. The corollary here is that the process must allow the board and its advisers sufficient time to gather all the information they need to arrive at an informed and reasoned decision. Thus, you should avoid efforts by managers or prospective partners or buyers to impose artificial deadlines on your decision-making process.

Making decisions about your hospital's future in reaction to crises is never a good idea. Forcing important decisions into artificially short time frames curbs the ability of your board and your advisers to adequately investigate the problems. As the fiduciaries charged with the duty to exercise due care over charitable assets, you must make not only the ultimate decision but also a reasoned decision. If you do not, you expose yourself unnecessarily to personal liability for any losses sustained by your charity during the conversion.

Conclusion

Strategic planning for your hospital's future should be an ongoing process of your board. If you are planning for the possibility of conversion, your planning should begin with the goals you hope to achieve. Once your goals are determined, you will be able to assess the viability of the variety of options open to you. If you do not engage in appropriate strategic planning, your conversion decision may well be forced on you, which can seriously impair your ability to protect your charity's assets during the process. If your charity suffers losses as a result, you will face personal exposure to significant liability for those losses. We think your choice is clear. Plan carefully and protect your charity. That will protect you.

3

Planning for the
Post-Conversion Charity

The decision to convert your hospital cannot properly be made without simultaneously planning for the post-conversion period. If you attempt to postpone decision making in this area until after the deal closes, you invite unwelcome surprises in the form of unforseen legal problems, community hostility, and an inability to carry out any charitable mission on a timely basis.

It is, therefore, important that, as part of the strategic-planning process, you recognize a few simple facts. First, the decision to convert your hospital means that you are creating a new reality: you are no longer going to be responsible for operating a community hospital, you are going to be in the grant-making business. This new entity requires new skills, new structures, and different types of advisers than you required previously.

Second, the law of *cy pres* (explained below) places significant restrictions on how you can spend the conversion proceeds, and these restrictions may conflict with both your goals and your community's expectations. It will, therefore, be necessary for you not only to create a spending plan that complies with these legal restrictions but also to educate your community and bring it into the decision-making process. Your failure to take these steps will almost certainly create problems as you proceed to develop a spending plan for the conversion proceeds.

And, finally, upon close of the transaction, you will likely have far more money than you previously had in endowment accounts. You need to be prepared for this added responsibility by retaining investment advisers and creating financial systems with increased capacity.

Table 3.1 provides an overview of post-conversion goals and the new structures and advisers that are necessary.

Goal 1: Educate the Affected Community and Involve It in the Decision-Making Process

We discussed this issue at some length in the previous chapter and will not repeat those comments here. However, it should be mentioned that developing an effective method of educating the pub-

Table 3.1. Goals and structures of the post-conversion foundation

Post-Conversion Goals	New Structures	Advisers
1. Educate your community and involve it in the process	Community advisory committees, focus groups	Community groups, health consultants
2. Create a corporate structure that complies with state law	Revised mission statement, restated articles of incorporation	Legal counsel
3. Create a charitable spending plan for the post-conversion foundation	New trust documents, endowment funds	Legal counsel
4. Develop an investment and financial-management plan	Written investment guidelines, financial-oversight plan	Financial manager

lic about the transaction from the earliest stages will go a long way toward blunting criticism. When the decision to convert is based on a careful and considered judgment regarding the continued financial viability of the hospital, it is important to communicate that judgment to the community. Reasoned decisions are generally understood and well received by the community, even if they entail a certain amount of uncertainty and concern about the future.

It will also be essential to advise the community of the legal restrictions that attach to the proceeds. The mandated use restrictions should be explained to the community before the conversion so that expectations and reality coincide. The community will generally view the spending plan for the proceeds as its quid pro quo for the sale of the hospital. Because the community will be the beneficiary of the trust created from the conversion proceeds, you must win community support for your charitable-uses plan, and failing to advise the community of the restrictions that apply is a sure way to lose that support.

Goal 2: Create a Structure for the Post-Conversion Charity That Is Consistent with Your State Law

A key issue that needs to be addressed is the structure of the entity that will manage the assets of the new charity and carry out its mission. In some states, the law dictates the available options. However, in most states, the decision is left to the board of directors of the converting hospital. You have many choices for the structure of the entity that will survive the sale of your hospital, including these:

- Retain the existing corporate structure and board with a new mission statement and new corporate purpose.

- Transfer the proceeds to a successor nonprofit hospital (or hospitals).

- Transfer the proceeds to an existing grant-making foundation.
- Create a new community-based foundation.

Which structure is most appropriate for your charity depends in large measure on your plans for the use of the conversion proceeds.

In our experience, the most common choice is simply to leave the board of the corporation that owned the hospital in place with the new mission of administering the endowment that results from the conversion (as well as any other retained assets). Leaving the old hospital board in charge of the sale endowment is the most common choice for obvious reasons. The board members naturally feel that they still have a role to play in serving the community. Administering a charity plan funded with millions of dollars is an attractive vehicle for that purpose. However, three potential problems should be considered. First, the board probably has not had previous experience managing large investment pools. The risk here is that investment mistakes will be made for which the board members may be personally liable if they do not take appropriate steps to secure adequate professional advice. Second, the board may have to spend significant amounts of money designing a charitable-uses plan that will satisfy state law and comply with its charitable charter. Simply transferring the conversion proceeds to another nonprofit hospital or to an existing community foundation avoids this cost. Third, the board will probably need to create a new administrative structure to assist it in its new mission. This new management will cost money that could be saved by using the existing and experienced staff of a community foundation. So before you just assume that the old board should retain control of the endowment and the future charitable mission of the surviving entity, give careful thought to whether other organizations or structures are better suited to the task.

The second option is to use another nonprofit community hospital as the successor trustee for the conversion proceeds. This option is the "purest" under trust law as the successor organization is likely the most similar to the converted hospital in mission and community served. Moreover it is also important to keep in mind that because most nonprofit hospitals are dedicated to providing hospital services to their communities by the terms of their corporate charters, some hospital-related purpose may well be imposed on the surviving charity by the state regulatory agency reviewing your transaction. The California attorney general has taken a strong stand in requiring that nonprofit hospital assets continue to be used for those same hospital purposes after conversion. Such views, if shared by the appropriate authority in your state, should cause the board to at least consider the option of selecting another nonprofit hospital as the successor trustee of the conversion proceeds.

There are, in fact, several advantages to this option. No new administrative structure is needed, and the sale proceeds can be turned over to the management of one or more nonprofit hospitals serving your community. Whether the funds are to be restricted to particular uses is a matter for the board to decide. In addition, no funds need to be spent devising a new charitable-uses program, which can mean significant savings.

A third structural option is to give the conversion proceeds to a local foundation experienced in managing restricted charitable trusts. The funds can be given to such a foundation with detailed restrictions on allowable expenditures or with a broad health mandate if that is permitted under your state's trust law. In a transaction in California, a board sold its hospital, leaving a $50 million endowment. The board decided that it did not want responsibility for managing such a large fund and administering a grant-making charitable program—a decision grounded partly in the recognition that the board had no experience doing either. The board decided to develop a charitable program designed to accomplish specific goals, including these:

- Supporting the major nonprofit hospitals serving its community

- Providing a health-insurance program for uninsured children residing within its community

- Funding needed community-benefit programs

Suitable trust documents were created, and discussions commenced about implementing this plan by turning the endowment fund over to a large, experienced community foundation to invest and manage in a way consistent with the preestablished goals. This decision was made to satisfy community concerns over the use of this large endowment, which the community viewed as its money. This decision also satisfied California trust law because the funds were dedicated to the same purposes and to the same community that had been served by the old hospital.

Finally, the board can create a new community-based foundation to manage and disburse the conversion proceeds. This is the option generally preferred by local community groups, and it has been incorporated into proposed legislation sponsored by consumer-advocacy groups. It has the disadvantage of incurring all the costs inherent in the creation of any new corporation but has the advantage of allowing, at least in theory, the most community input, especially in the selection of a new board of directors.

In choosing one structure or another, you need to remember that you are still fiduciaries. Your choice should not be based on personal benefit. The fact that your board wants to remain in control of the endowment fund is not reason enough for that to be the choice. You should carefully consider all alternatives and document the reasons for your ultimate selection. If you have based your choice on what is best for your community, you should have no problems.

Goal 3: Create a Charitable-Spending Plan for Your Post-Conversion Foundation

Assuming that you have decided to retain control over your post-conversion assets and not simply transfer them to a successor nonprofit entity, you will need to create a charitable-spending plan. Whatever structure you use to house your endowment, you are still trustees of assets that are dedicated to particular charitable purposes. Those purposes are defined by your nonprofit hospital's corporate documents and its historical operations. The fact that you have sold that hospital and will have a new structure to operate from does not change the trust on which the conversion proceeds are held.

Key Tip! The allowable uses of your post-conversion proceeds are defined by a legal doctrine called the *cy pres* rule. Taken from the Norman French and meaning "as close as possible," this rule requires that your post-conversion use of the transaction proceeds be as similar as possible to your preconversion use. This rule generally requires that the funds be used for hospital and related medical purposes.

What is included in your spending plan will depend on the scope of the charitable charter under which you operated your hospital. It will also depend on the scope of the activities you conducted through your hospital system. Finally, it will depend on what you want to accomplish within the discretionary constraints imposed by trust law.

Although some states approach spending plans differently, California has developed three specific legal options:

- Historical-services option
- Charitable-component option
- Supporting-organization option

The Historical-Services Option

The historical-services approach attempts to replicate, through grant making, the historical services provided by the hospital prior to conversion. It essentially defines the charitable trust using two criteria: the historical services provided by the preconversion hospital and the primary service area of the preconversion hospital.

The first criterion is established by measuring the historical expenditures of the hospital for various categories of services—for example, acute-care inpatient services, outpatient services, community-benefit programs, preventive health programs, and educational services. Once expenditures are divided among categories, each category receives a percentage of the annual post-conversion income commensurate with its historical share of preconversion expenditures.

The second criterion—the primary service area of the hospital—ensures that you serve the same beneficiaries. You can determine this area by conducting an analysis of the patient census-tract information for the years immediately preceding conversion. In California, we have defined a hospital's primary service area by zip code. Primary service areas can also be defined by other methods. Generally, services funded by the post-conversion foundation are thereafter limited to residents of the neighborhoods previously within the hospital's primary service area.

Two other conditions are also normally included in this model. First, because the converting entity was a nonprofit charitable corporation, grants are restricted to other nonprofit charitable corporations (or governmental institutions) serving the primary service area. One exception has been the funding of medical and hospital insurance for the medically indigent residing in the primary service area. The choice of providers for such insurance has not been limited to nonprofit companies but rather has been made on the most cost-effective basis.

The second condition involves a recognition that historical program categories can become obsolete; technological innovations may permit services that were once provided on an inpatient basis to be provided on an outpatient basis. Because this trend is escalating, converting charities in California have been permitted to use a cost-of-living type adjustment to reallocate funds from inpatient to outpatient services based on industry data showing changes in utilization rates.

Because this option involves the change from an operating charity to a grant-making charity, it has been the position of the California attorney general's office that it requires court approval.

Normally, the court is petitioned to approve restated articles of incorporation that establish the conditions set forth above as nonamendable articles or bylaws. The board then has a court-approved set of rules by which to operate.

In essence, this option provides basic guidelines for expenditures—by historical service category, beneficiary class, and grant recipient. Within these general rules, the board has complete discretion to direct the charitable funds. Although it is not required, we strongly recommend that the board engage consultants and conduct community focus groups to define community needs and then establish spending priorities within the trust restrictions consistent with those needs.

The Charitable-Component Option

A second approach defines the charitable components of the hospital's past operations and then permits the sale proceeds to be used to continue funding those same charitable components at other nonprofit or governmental hospitals serving the same community. Instead of measuring all historical hospital services, this model seeks to limit future funding to categories of past services that were uniquely charitable, as distinguished from commercial. Examples include uncompensated charity care, immunization programs, community-benefit programs, education, research, and teaching.

Each component is identified and its percentage of the whole defined based on relative historical funding. Separate endowment funds are then created for each component, and the income from those funds is used to support ongoing services. As in the historical-services approach, restrictions are placed on providers and service areas, and a cost-of-living type adjustment among the categories is included to reflect ongoing changes in medical delivery systems.

Also like the historical-services option, this approach requires court approval and the creation of an enforceable trust document containing the appropriate restrictions on use. The board then has clear guidance on the ways it may use the post-conversion funds and the discretion to expend the endowment-fund income, provided it complies with the terms of the trust.

Again, we strongly recommend that the board engage consultants and obtain community input to determine community needs and create a charitable program that meets those needs.

The Supporting-Organization Option

An option that blends the outright gift of the sale proceeds to other nonprofit hospitals serving the same community and the approaches described above is the supporting-organization approach. (A supporting organization is a technical form of a private foundation under the Internal Revenue Code that permits a grant-making foundation to avoid the distribution restrictions of the private foundation. See Internal Revenue Code, § 509(a)(3).) Here, the surviving charity agrees to utilize its sale proceeds to support programs carried out at other nonprofit hospitals serving the same community.

Because all the sale proceeds will be used for hospital-related purposes, the California attorney general's office has treated this model favorably. The supporting organization can take the assets with almost no restrictions except for geographical service area. This model maximizes program flexibility but limits the fund recipients to other hospitals.

Goal 4: Establish an Investment and Management Structure for the Conversion Proceeds

Now that you have sold your hospital and have, ideally, a sizable amount of cash instead, what do you with the money? The answer takes us back to your basic fiduciary duties: you must manage the assets of your charity prudently. You are not responsible for operating a community hospital anymore. You are now an investment manager—a job that, in all probability, is new to you. In order to fulfill your fiduciary responsibilities in this job, you need to take the following steps:

1. Define your investment goals

2. Select a qualified investment adviser

3. Establish written investment guidelines

4. Monitor investment performance

5. Negotiate terms to protect your charity from loss and excessive fees

Step 1: Setting Your Investment Goals

When thinking about your investment goals, keep in mind that the board is now a long-term investor that will have to earn sufficient income to grow and to support its ongoing charitable programs. This does not mean that you should decide on how large a program to have and then set your investment goals to achieve that level of income. Just the opposite is more appropriate. You need to set your program expenditures at levels that are achievable with reasonable investment objectives.

What are reasonable investment objectives? We will not pretend to tell you how to allocate assets among various types of investment instruments. However, having certain broad investment objectives is crucial if you are to comply with fiduciary obligations. These are among those objectives:

- Managing your investments in a manner that yields sufficient income to carry out your charitable program

- Keeping your investments sufficiently liquid so that you can get to your assets if you need them

- Ensuring reasonable capital growth over the long term

- Creating an investment portfolio that is appropriate for a long-term investor, including diversification, return on investment, and prudent levels of risk

This last objective has two requirements. First, you must try to earn market rates of return on your investments given an appropriate degree of risk. Second, you must invest safely, keeping in mind your charity's programmatic needs. Both sound easy, but can be difficult to implement. A simple example may illustrate the point. An investor who placed all his or her assets in ninety-day U.S. Treasury bills between 1974 and 1994 would have earned an annualized return of 7.2 percent—a good, safe investment. However, when adjusted for inflation over that same period, the real return was only 1.7 percent. That rate of return would almost certainly subject fiduciaries to serious criticism for failing to create a balanced and diversified investment portfolio. You thus need to walk a fine line between risk and safety in managing your investments. To do so, you have to know how to screen investment advisers in order to select one who best suits your investment strategies and goals.

Step 2: Selecting an Investment Adviser

Once you get past the brothers-in-law of board members and your chair's long-lost cousin, the list of investment advisers to choose from is still enormous. What do you look for? First and foremost, the adviser you choose must understand and appreciate the rules governing fiduciary investments so that you can minimize your own liability as a fiduciary. Indeed, the firm or firms you choose must be willing to assume fiduciary responsibility to your charity as a manager of its investments. If a firm is unwilling to assume this responsibility, reject it out of hand. Look for firms that have a record of providing advice to other nonprofit endowments or large ERISA (Employee Retirement Income Security Act) retirement funds. Firms that provide investment advice to retirement funds governed by ERISA are required by federal law to act as fiduciaries and bear the risk that entails (ERISA, §§ 409, 502).

In fact, the statutory standards imposed on investment advisors by ERISA, although not required by trust law, are useful guides for trustees in evaluating various firms. For example, if the administra-

tors of an ERISA retirement plan hire investment advisers, those advisers are required (1) to follow the plan's written investment-
policy statement, which must address asset-allocation decisions,
investment strategies, and specific investment objectives; (2) to analyze and advise the plan administrator about the risk of each investment decision relative to its return; (3) to diversify the plan's
investments; (4) to select specific investment managers according to
prudence standards set out in the statute; (5) to monitor investments
regularly; and (6) to prepare regular evaluations of investments and
report to plan administrators and participants. If the plan administrators hire investment advisers who comply with these requirements, ERISA exempts the administrators from any liability for acts
or omissions of the investment advisers in making investment decisions (ERISA, P.L. 93-406, Title II, § 405, 29 U.S.C. § 1105(d)).

These standards give a good idea of the types of services trustees
can seek from investment advisors. Will the firm you are considering assist the board in developing written guidelines for its investment policies and objectives? What kind of experience does the firm
have, and what will it do to assist the board in evaluating the risk
of various types of investment instruments? What kind of research
capability does the firm have? What is its performance history in
managing the kinds of assets the board feels comfortable with?
What kind of plan does the firm recommend for diversifying proposed investments? Will the firm diversify its selection of investment managers and provide the board with regular quantitative and
qualitative reports about the results achieved by each? What kind
of process does the firm have to monitor investments on an ongoing
basis? How often will the firm provide written reports to the board
showing the performance of your investment portfolio? What kind
of and how much liability insurance does the firm carry? What are
its fees?

A key focus of the board should be the *experience* of the invest-
ment-manager candidates in managing the types of investments the
board feels most comfortable with. Not all firms have the capability

or desire to provide the complete array of increasingly complex investment opportunities that exist. Once you have settled on investment objectives and guidelines, make sure that the firm that manages your investments has experience with all the types of investments your board wants to consider. Or hire a firm to oversee a group of investment managers who have the requisite capability. Do not risk your assets to provide a learning curve for novices.

You should compare the *research capabilities* of the firms you are considering. Do they have the experience and the wherewithal to discover needed information about prospective investments? Do they provide recommendations based on their research in a format that you can understand? Remember, your investment decisions, even when made on the advice of experts, must be reasonable. If you do not understand the advice you are receiving, you will not be able to defend your decisions.

You should check the *results* achieved by each candidate in managing investments of the type your board wants to make. Everyone will tell you that past performance is no guarantee of future results. That is true. But comparing investment results by managers of different asset classes over the same time periods does indicate their relative abilities. You should not ignore that information. Moreover, do not rely solely on the investment returns achieved over some period of time by the various firms. The level of return is only half the equation. The other half is risk. What degree of risk did a particular firm take to achieve the returns it secured? Was the client adequately compensated for the degree of risk the investment manager was assuming with its assets? These are important questions that you must address. Modern portfolio theory provides several methods for quantifying the level of risk taken by investment managers with particular instruments. You need to make sure that the degree of risk being recommended is prudent given your investment objectives and that the expected returns adequately compensate your charity for the risk being taken.

Step 3: Establishing Written Investment
Guidelines That Include Diversification

Each firm you consider should be asked whether it can assist in developing written investment guidelines for the board to follow. Written investment guidelines serve two important functions. First, they force the board to actively consider what investment policies and strategies best suit the needs of the board and the charitable program it intends to carry out. Second, written guidelines bring discipline to the board's review of particular investment recommendations, whether they are made directly to the board or to management. These reviews provide ongoing measures of the investment performance of the charity's investment advisers. Often called "investment-policy statements," these written guidelines can and should be quite specific. They can, for example, list the specific asset classes the charity will invest in and the percentage of funds to be invested within each class. They can set performance guidelines that the investment managers must meet to retain the business of the charity. Remember, you are the client. You should insist that your investment values and goals guide the investment manager's decisions.

The duty of due care also suggests that one of the board's investment strategies should be to diversify its investments to spread risk. Several types of diversification should be considered. At the most basic level, the board should consider diversifying its investments among more than one investment manager. A large endowment may exceed the insurance limits of some or perhaps all investment houses. If this is the case, the board should at least ask whether it is prudent to place more funds in the hands of a particular manager than that manager can protect with insurance.

Apart from the insurance issue, the board may feel that having more than one manager promotes safety and improved performance by fostering competition in both areas. The board might consider whether it should retain one firm to provide fiduciary oversight of two or more fund managers. Firms that provide such services may be in a better position than members of the board to evaluate the strengths and weaknesses of firms offering investment services. Such firms can provide continuing oversight and reports to the board concerning the management of the portfolio. Such reporting will assist the board in measuring the results of particular fund managers against the investment guidelines the board has adopted and provide a record of the board's decision-making process.

The board should also consider diversifying the types of investments it makes. Different firms will recommend different mixes of stocks, bonds, mutual funds, and a variety of other types of instruments. Some firms may recommend diversification in international markets. Ultimately, the board will have to choose from among the recommendations made by investment advisors. Again, those choices should be informed by written guidelines adopted by the board in advance.

Step 4: Monitoring Investment Performance

The board should take steps to ensure ongoing oversight. Whether that function is handled directly by the board, by a committee of the board, or by professional advisers is a choice you have to make. Even if your board chooses to place investment responsibility in a single firm, you must oversee the work of that firm. Therefore, the board must think about what kind of reports it wants to receive from its investment advisers and about how it will use the reports it does receive to assess results.

Step 5: Negotiating Terms to Protect the
Charity from Loss or Excessive Fees

One key variable to consider in hiring investment advisers is the *extent and nature of the liability insurance* they carry to protect themselves and their clients. If you are entrusting millions of dollars to an investment firm, assuming you decide that some sort of custodial accounts are appropriate, you want to make sure that the custodian has theft and negligence insurance for each deposit you make. Most firms will have such coverage, but you should insist that it be a contractual component of your relationship. All licensed securities dealers are covered by the basic insurance provided by the Securities Investors Protection Corporation (SIPC). That insurance is limited to $500,000 in losses. Most major investment houses have significant private insurance well above the SIPC minimum. Typically, for large institutional investors, coverage is provided for investments up to $50 million. You need to find out what insurance the firms you are considering carry and what kinds of losses are covered. The failure to secure available insurance protection could be considered negligence if your charity suffers a loss. You will be on the hook personally if that occurs.

The *fees* you will pay for investment services are always negotiable. The customary fee structure is based on a percentage of the assets under management. Such arrangements, if market-based, are appropriate. Compensation arrangements with investment advisers are regulated under federal law, in particular the Investment Advisors Act of 1940 (15 U.S.C. §§ 80b-1 et seq.). You want to avoid any arrangements that may create perverse incentives for the investment manager. In particular, you do not want to give the manager compensation incentives that encourage highly risky investments that, although likely to achieve large returns and thereby to increase the manager's fees, place your assets at too great a risk of loss. Whatever arrangements you are comfortable with, get competitive bids. That will protect you against overpaying.

Conclusion

Planning your charity's future is an exciting opportunity. The constraints are your charitable charter, state law, and your fiduciary obligations. If you create a process designed to satisfy your duties, you will enjoy the excitement of the opportunity.

4

Selling Your Hospital

This chapter looks at what happens when a nonprofit board, after careful consideration of all relevant issues, decides to sell its hospital to a for-profit buyer. That sale is a "conversion." When we use the phrase *hospital conversion,* we are describing a transaction that results in the transfer of ownership or control over hospital assets from a nonprofit corporation to a for-profit company. Sales, joint ventures, some types of leases, and even management agreements can all result in the conversion of nonprofit assets. The two most prevalent conversion transactions are the sale and the joint venture. This chapter will deal with the outright sale of a nonprofit hospital.

The key requirements for trustees in every sale transaction are tied directly to the core fiduciary duties. For the duty of obedience to purpose, the key requirement is developing a conversion plan that satisfies the hospital's charitable purpose. For the duty of due care, the requirement is to assure that fair market value is received for the hospital assets. And for the duty of loyalty, it is guaranteeing that there are no conflicts of interest in the sale process.

Meeting all these requirements may not be a simple task. For example, with respect to the duty of obedience to charitable purpose, unless your state law authorizes the trustees to sell all or substantially all of their charity's assets, you may be precluded from converting the hospital altogether. And even where such a legal right exists, it is always difficult for trustees to develop a post-conversion plan that is consistent with the charity's preconversion articles of incorporation and historical uses. After all, the board no longer operates a community hospital, and the creation of an appropriate charitable-uses (spending) plan, as we discussed in Chapter Two, is essential to comply with this duty. The duty of due care requires that trustees obtain fair market value for their hospital and raises similar challenges. Generally, the market should dictate the price. Valuations and fairness opinions (explained below) are poor substitutes for the market in establishing value, and failure to convince regulatory authorities that you have obtained fair market value brings with it a significant risk of personal liability. Finally, the duty of loyalty requires that board members ensure against conflicts of interest at all levels. Trustees may not enrich themselves at the charity's expense; management that is advising the board should not receive financial advantages from the sale; and the experts the board retains should not have business ties to the buyer. These three basic requirements should guide the process to sell your hospital, and only by meeting them can a board comply with its fiduciary obligations.

The Sale Process

The simplest form of conversion is an outright sale. It is simple from the regulators' point of view because it eliminates many of the difficult issues that are raised by arrangements that envision an ongoing business relationship between the nonprofit entity and the for-profit acquirer. It is simple from the seller's point of view for the same reasons. A sale is by far the easiest of the conversion transactions to complete and carries the least risk for the board.

If your nonprofit board decides that a sale is in the best interests of the hospital and its beneficiaries, then three words that you should have in mind at all times are process, process, and process. The right process is the best assurance of a good result: the hospital and its directors emerge from the conversion with their goals met, with the support of their community, and without legal liabilities. Here is an outline of that process:

1. Select the right experts to market and price your hospital.
2. Negotiate reasonable fee agreements:
   A. Get competitive bids.
   B. Define the specific tasks you want performed.
3. Protect against possible conflicts of interest:
   A. Identify potential management conflicts.
   B. Identify your experts' ties with potential buyers.
4. Understand the valuation advice you receive:
   A. Understand the difference between "fair" and "fair market value."
   B. Understand the difference between fairness opinions and valuation analysis.
   C. Learn the strengths and weaknesses of the three key valuation methodologies (discounted cash flow, comparable companies, and similar transactions) and ask the right questions.
   D. Know the legal standards you are required to meet.
5. Establish a proper marketing plan:
   A. Develop a request for proposals to market your hospital.
   B. Establish criteria for evaluating offers.
   C. Maximize the number of potential buyers.
   D. Create an auction or "back to the market" process.
   E. Select the best offer.
6. Document the deal properly:
   A. Make sure the letter of intent is clear.
   B. Create a pro forma financial statement to make sure all sale contingencies are understood by the board.
   C. Use great care in reviewing the definitive agreements; once they are signed, your hospital is gone.

7. Most important, make sure you understand what your experts are telling you and decide whether it makes sense. These people work for you; make them explain their conclusions until you are comfortable with the answers.

Getting the Right Advice at the Right Price

The first step in creating the right process is to hire the right experts to guide you through it. The need for experts should be self-evident. How many hospitals have you sold? The answer, in all probability, is none. For-profit acquirers, however, usually have bought many hospitals.

The most obvious risk of failing to hire the necessary experts is that you will be personally liable for selling the hospital below its fair market value. The first rule of selling your nonprofit hospital is that you must get fair market value for the assets. If you do not, you cost your community substantial money; you diminish the amount of health services you will be able to provide in the future; and, of no small import, you expose board members to personal liability for the difference between the price secured and the fair market value of the assets sold. Because hospitals are not normally sold for small change, these costs can be high indeed!

Fair market value is, in the context of a sale, a fairly simple term to define. It is the most likely price that would be received in a sale between a willing buyer and a willing seller where neither is under any undue pressure. It follows that the surest way to secure fair market value for your assets is to sell them on the open market, where they are exposed to as many willing and able buyers as possible. In fact, the nonprofit board should attempt to create a sale process that will get the most potential buyers interested in your hospital.

Selling hospitals is not like selling cars or even houses, where there may be hundreds of potential buyers and dozens if not hundreds of competing products. The odds are quite high that your hospital will be the only one available for sale in your community and perhaps even in a large geographical region. It is also probable that the number of potential buyers will be small, possibly only one. It may be difficult for the selling board to know what the asking price should be or even how to go about finding buyers and marketing the hospital, and for this reason the use of appropriate experts is necessary.

Marketing and Valuation Experts

The first questions that boards should ask in making the decision to sell a nonprofit hospital are, What should the asking price be? and How should the hospital be marketed? Answering these two questions may call for advice from different types of experts. The right asking price can be determined by valuation firms or by firms with expertise in selling hospitals, usually investment bankers; the marketing issues can be addressed only by firms with experience in selling hospitals. Boards often consider hiring the same firm to provide the initial valuation opinion and also to market and sell the hospital. There is no clear best way; the choice of consultants and advisers should reflect the particular situation confronting your board.

Hiring the same firm that provides the initial valuation to also market and sell the hospital can save money because that firm may discount its valuation fee to secure the opportunity to earn the fees associated with selling the facility. Moreover, the firm that does the initial valuation will learn a great deal about the facility being sold. This knowledge should translate into lower costs in selling the facility, which can save the hospital money.

The downside to using the same firm for both tasks is that the firm may have an incentive to undervalue the assets. Most investment-banking firms have a "success-based" fee structure, by which they receive a percentage of the sale price for finding a buyer. Underpricing the hospital slightly may increase the likelihood of a sale without substantially decreasing the sales commission. It may cost you several million dollars, but it guarantees their fee. Moreover, the board loses the opportunity to have the check and second opinion that using two firms would provide.

Using one firm to provide the initial valuation and another to market the hospital also has advantages and disadvantages. One of the major advantages is that the valuation firm has no incentive to undervalue or overvalue the assets being sold. The firm's fee will be unaffected by extraneous concerns. As noted above, this approach also provides the nonprofit board with a second opinion on valuation because the firm hired to market and sell the hospital will also likely have valuation experience. The value of obtaining a second opinion should not be ignored by the members of a nonprofit board, who face personal exposure for a sale at less than fair market value. A second opinion is especially valuable when there are few buyers— or perhaps only one buyer—interested in the hospital. With multiple bidders, valuations are far less important because the market itself will determine value.

The principal disadvantage of using two firms to value and market a hospital is the increased cost of two separate contracts when neither contractor can offer to lower fees for the opportunity to do both tasks. In addition, transaction costs are associated with both hiring the firms and dealing with potential buyers. Using two firms will probably increase the transaction costs on both fronts. Negotiating the terms of two contracts for expert advice is more costly than negotiating one. Also, costs are associated with gathering and presenting information to potential buyers. Because the information that buyers need in order to decide whether and how much to bid is quite similar to the information that experts need to value the hospital properly, using two firms duplicates effort. How much it costs and whether the additional cost is justified by other factors is a business judgment the board has to make.

Key Tip! Properly documenting the decisions made when hiring experts will provide the board with a paper trail showing that it has acted responsibly and met its duty of due care.

The process of selecting appropriate experts to advise the nonprofit board should set the tone for the other processes necessary for completing the sale of a hospital. Keep in mind at all times that the hospital probably represents the vast bulk of your charity's assets and that you will get only one chance to sell it. That consideration should lead you to take the same care in selecting experts to advise you as you will take in the other steps of the sale process.

Negotiating Expert Fees

Experts cost money, sometimes serious money. Accordingly, the nonprofit board must carefully negotiate appropriate arrangements to retain the expert advice it needs. Here too the market is the board's best friend, so get competitive bids from qualified firms for whatever advice the board wants.

The fee structure should reflect the specific services you are buying. For example, flat fees are generally more suitable for valuation opinions, but percentage fees are common for the marketing of hospitals. You would not use a percentage fee structure for valuation opinions because that would skew the outcome upward almost every time. By contrast, you want the marketing firm's fee structure to create an incentive to obtain a higher price, and the percentage fee does that.

You may wish to consider incentive payments for marketing fees when there are relatively few potential buyers. Such incentives will tend to offset the marketing firm's desire to get a quick sale agreement to ensure receipt of the fee (which is typically contingent on the close of a sale transaction). Obviously, the larger the incentives the greater the effect on the marketing firm's efforts. Sliding-scale incentives might be considered as well. For example, the marketing firm can be offered a relatively low fixed percentage of the sale price up to the initial valuation figure you have received. But you might offer increasingly higher percentage fees on amounts exceeding the initial valuation. Such incentive payments will encourage the marketing firm to replicate as closely as possible the results that would be expected in an auction with many qualified buyers. The fee structure you decide to use should be consistent with the market in your area.

Once you have received proposals that are comparable, you can determine the bidders that are best suited to the board's needs.

Avoiding Conflicts of Interest

Once you have retained a firm to value and market the assets, the next step is to create the process for selling the hospital. That process will undoubtedly involve your hospital's top managers because they will have most of the knowledge about the facility that both the marketing firm and potential buyers will need. Moreover, our experience shows that most nonprofit boards rely a great deal on the business judgment of their management, which is appropriate for this most important decision. However, equally important, the board needs to realize that senior managers may have serious potential conflicts of interest in the sale process. For example, they may want to keep their same jobs with the purchasing company, or they may be opposed to the sale because they fear losing their jobs.

Key Tip! The first task in setting up a sale process is to protect against conflicts of interest. If the information you base your judgment on is biased, your chances of reaching the right decision are substantially reduced.

Several steps can be taken to minimize or eliminate the potential adverse effects of conflicts of interest on the part of managers or others. The board can appoint a committee of experienced businesspersons from the board to have primary responsibility for conducting negotiations. Or the board may prefer to hire independent consultants to conduct the negotiations or, at a minimum, to review the actions of senior management in this process.

Conflicts of interest involving the experts the board retains are also a major concern. Investment-banking firms often have close business ties with the for-profit companies most likely to be potential buyers for your hospital. They may have represented them in other hospital transactions, securities offerings, or other types of transactions. The desire to handle future matters for the for-profit buyer may color the advice that the firm provides to you, and you need to be aware of that conflict. For example, if the firm you retain provides an analysis of potential buyers that ranks one far above the others for reasons that seem counterintuitive, treat that ranking as a red flag. Find out whether the firms have a business relationship or any other facts that might suggest a conflict of interest on the part of the investment banker. There is no particular reason in a straight cash sale for an investment-banking firm to favor one buyer over another for reasons other than price. These firms are, after all, not health-quality experts, but simply sales and marketing firms.

However, investment bankers may appropriately advise you that, for competitive reasons, your hospital is likely to have greater value to one potential buyer than to others. Indeed, this type of advice is precisely the reason you hire investment bankers. However, that advice is not a reason to exclude other potential bidders from the process. Your first rule in the bidding process should be "the more the merrier!"

In the valuation process, you may get offers from the valuation consulting groups of one or more of the national accounting firms. Those firms may represent the large for-profit companies interested in acquiring your hospital. You should know whether they do before you retain them to provide you with valuation advice. The national accounting firms that also have valuation consulting groups may have the ability to create "Chinese walls" to separate the valuation work they offer to do for you from accounting work they do with potential buyers. But you should be aware of the issue, know the facts, and examine carefully any proposals from firms that also do accounting work for potential buyers. Other things being equal, we would not recommend hiring a firm with such ties to potential buyers where alternatives are readily available.

Key Tip! Requiring full disclosure from all potential investment bankers or valuation firms of financial ties to potential buyers is necessary to protect against conflicts of interest.

The key point is that the board needs to be aware of all potential conflicts among those providing advice to it concerning a transaction. The board needs to address those conflicts and document its process for dealing with them, so there can be no question about the board's good-faith reliance on the advice it has received.

The board must also take steps to avoid conflicts of interest among its own members. If members of your board are involved in businesses that are affiliated with or that transact significant business with the hospital, you need to make sure that those board members are not using the sale of the hospital to gain personal advantage for themselves. For example, doctors who serve on your board may own interests in labs or medical practices that meet the needs of your hospital's patients. Those businesses may be attractive to potential buyers. You should assure yourselves that no such considerations are influencing those board members' consideration of or voting on the sale of the hospital. Make sure you require disclosure of such potential areas of conflict by all board members when you begin even to consider sale or conversion of your hospital. If any potential conflicts arise, have your counsel advise the board on the best way to deal with them. Remember, the existence of any self-dealing in these transactions automatically changes the fiduciary standard to which you are held from the prudent person standard to the self-dealing standards, which are typically more difficult to satisfy.

Obtaining a Formal Valuation

Once the decision to sell your hospital is made and a valuation or investment-banking firm is retained to advise you about pricing, you have to decide whether you need a formal valuation opinion or fairness opinion. If you do, you then have to decide when to obtain such an opinion, from whom, and at what cost.

Necessity

The decision about obtaining a formal valuation depends, in large part, on the sale process you are using. When you are able to create an active market for your hospital, with multiple bidders and price competition, we question the practical value of such opinions. They are, after all, merely an estimate of the price the market would place on the hospital. When the market is allowed to work, it will provide that price in the bids received. In the end, your hospital is worth what potential buyers are willing to pay for it, not what some expert thinks they might pay for it. In California, we have, therefore, generally downplayed the need for such opinions, especially in auction sales that produce multiple bids. Our view is that such opinions add little to the process in such circumstances and are not worth their substantial cost.

Sometimes an auction either is not possible because there is only one buyer or is not desired by the charitable corporation. In fact, in some situations, a nonprofit hospital may pursue an exclusive marketing strategy targeting a single most likely buyer. This strategy might be employed, for example, to avoid giving competitors (who are not likely buyers) access to competitive information through due diligence reviews. In this situation, there is no market validation of the sale price, and, therefore, a valuation or fairness opinion may well be necessary as part of the selling hospital board's due care review. It may, in fact, be the only method that the board has available to demonstrate due care in the decision to sell the facility at the proposed price.

If you have decided that it is necessary to obtain a valuation or fairness opinion, you will need to answer three basic questions. When, from whom, and at what cost should you obtain such an opinion? The essential concern here is whether you are getting what you are paying for. We will deal with each of these questions.

Timing

When the valuation or fairness opinion is being used in lieu of an auction to validate a price without the benefit of competitive bids, the timing of the opinion is crucial. An opinion obtained before the sale is entered into has far greater credibility than one obtained after the fact, particularly when the opinion of value is provided by the investment-banking firm that is handling the sale of the hospital with a success-based fee structure. That firm's opinion is so seriously affected by its conflict of interest (its fee being subject to regulatory confirmation of the sale) that it is of questionable value. Presale acquisition of valuation information is simply logical from a due care standpoint.

It is our strong recommendation that if you intend to rely on an expert opinion (in lieu of a market-based auction) to defend your pricing decision, you should get that opinion (with all its supporting data and analysis) before you begin the process. You can then rely on that opinion throughout the process to meet your fiduciary obligation of due care.

Source and Cost

Next you need to decide who should provide the valuation or fairness opinion. Do you obtain that opinion from the same firm that you retained to handle the sale of the hospital, or do you use an independent firm? Without repeating our prior discussion, we would remind you that the trade-off is between credibility and the worth of a second opinion, on the one hand, and cost on the other. This is a decision you must make.

You should, however, keep in mind that although most states permit directors to rely on the opinion of experts, that reliance must be reasonable. When your expert is conflicted by a financial interest in the transaction and you are aware of that conflict, it adversely affects your ability to "reasonably" rely on that opinion. In essence, it creates an obligation on your part to closely examine that opinion before accepting it.

You also need to consider whether the cost savings generated by using a single expert is significant given the value of the deal. In a California case, the attorney general's office questioned the valuation report of an expert who we felt was conflicted. We obtained an independent valuation (at a reasonable price) and ended up negotiating a significant increase in sale price. It may well be that the

cost of obtaining an independent valuation opinion is not significant compared with the financial benefits that may be obtained.

Understanding Valuation Advice

You also need to consider the difference between an opinion normally provided by an investment-banking firm and that provided
by a valuation consultant. Although they use the same basic methodologies to reach their opinions, they generally phrase those opinions quite differently, and those differences may be significant in
obtaining regulatory approval depending on the law in your state.

Fairness Opinions and Valuation Opinions

Investment-banking firms generally provide what are called "fairness opinions"—formal, written opinions that the proposed transaction is "fair" to the seller. But these opinions are almost always
given after a buyer and seller have already agreed to a price. Although, generally, this form of opinion satisfies the corporate business judgment test (which is, of course, why it is has developed over
time), it will not suffice when the state statute requires a showing
that the price represents the fair market value.

The fairness opinion does not usually attempt to measure the
value of the asset to the buyer; rather, it indicates the investment value of the hospital to the seller. What does this mean in
plain English? When the sale price is below that designated as
"fair," the seller should not sell at all because the hospital is worth
more to it from an investment standpoint than the buyer is willing
to pay.

"Fair market value" is a different concept. It measures the most
likely price a willing buyer would pay for the hospital in a competitive situation. An opinion claiming to establish fair market value,
done properly, requires an examination of competitive factors. In
effect, it measures the likely investment value of the hospital to the
buyer, not the seller, and making such an estimate often requires

both the identification of likely buyers and an analysis of the amount those buyers would be likely to pay.

We will discuss this subject in detail later in this chapter. Here, it is important to note that (1) the terms *fair* and *fair market value* are not interchangeable and (2) fairness opinions generally will not meet the legal standard in states that require a showing of fair market value. Also, a fairness opinion will not protect board members at all when self-dealing is involved in those states that have adopted the "best deal in town" test (see the discussion of this test in Appendix B). This form of opinion does not even attempt to measure the likely sale price—let alone the best available sale price—and, therefore, fails to meet the statutory standard under this rule.

A board should, therefore, be sure that the opinion on which it relies (and for which it pays significant charitable funds) actually provides the legal "cover" it is seeking. One can imagine a board's consternation at having spent significant sums for a fairness opinion only to find out that it is legally insufficient. In the worst case, the board could find itself being sued both for failing to meet the requisite standard in establishing the sale price and for wasting charitable assets on a useless fairness opinion.

Although valuation consultants generally claim that they are providing an opinion of fair market value, as distinguished from a fairness opinion, they often use the same methodologies used by investment-banking firms. As a result, those estimates of fair market value will often fail to stand up under scrutiny.

To protect both your board and your charitable assets, you should take a few important steps:

- Have your attorneys determine the specific legal standard that you are required to meet. Have them draft an engagement letter with your expert that will provide you an opinion that meets that standard.

- Make sure that the experts you select are not conflicted by a financial relationship with the buyer; get a confirmation of that fact from them in writing.

- Read and carefully consider the expert's report before relying on it. Remember that although the law allows you to rely on experts' reports, such reliance must be reasonable. Reports from knowingly conflicted experts or reports that have obvious and apparent defects may not provide you the protection you are paying for— even when done by well-known firms.

Valuation Methodologies

Once you understand the types of opinions you are likely to receive from both investment-banking firms and valuation consultants, it is important as well to understand the substance of those reports— that is, the work product on which those opinions are based. Both types of firms tend to use the same valuation methodologies, and each of these methodologies has strengths and weaknesses. Having a general understanding of the type of analysis your experts are relying on not only will assist you in determining whether you are getting fair market value for your hospital but also will give you some insight into the type of expert you need and the work product you want that expert to produce. Generally, both types of firms use the same three methods of analysis: the discounted-cash-flow method, the comparable-companies method, and the similar-transaction method.

Discounted cash flow (DCF) is the method that most valuation experts believe is the most reliable in establishing value. Essentially it seeks to project future earnings over the near to mid-term by using past earnings, future management projections, or both as a guide. The experts then apply appropriate discount rates and calculate the present value of the projected income stream. An appropriate industry multiple is then applied to that income stream (discounted cash flow) and the result is an estimated value for the hospital.

This methodology accurately reflects the value of the hospital (as an investment) to the seller. Simply put, it is the expert's opinion of what the market would pay for that expected cash flow over time. What it does not measure is the value of the hospital to any specific buyer or the most likely price the hospital would bring in the open market. The reason is simple. Buyers will add into the calculation their best estimate of future earnings based on their perceptions of savings in purchasing costs and a host of other factors, or "synergies." That price is likely to be substantially higher than the hospital's own DCF projections. As an example, when an investor-owned hospital chain (or a nonprofit chain for that matter) has obtained substantial savings in its purchases of supplies and equipment through its enhanced buying power, these savings will directly affect the bottom line and increase profitability, thereby increasing the DCF they expect to produce from the hospital. Similarly, if the acquiring hospital chain has another hospital in close proximity to your hospital and if there are overlapping services, serious savings may be obtained by consolidating these services in a single location. Again, this consolidation should reduce costs and increase cash flows.

Key Tip! In every single case that we have looked at in California, the sale price of the hospital in the open market was substantially higher than the DCF value established by the hospital's experts, regardless of whether the expert was an investment banker or a valuation consultant.

In order to make the DCF analysis work in practice, it is essential to make it buyer-specific. Unfortunately, such an effort is likely to be expensive and time-consuming; consequently, most valuation and investment-banking firms would prefer to give you an off-the-shelf analysis that is inexpensive to produce and profitable for them. But it can be done. A buyer-specific analysis requires that your experts determine who the most likely buyers are (normally, a limited number of companies). Then they will need to identify the key synergies for each buyer and quantify them. These synergies will include such items as purchasing savings, consolidation of services, labor-cost reductions, and contractual advantages with providers. Although these factors will all be estimated, keep in mind that all the adjustments made by the experts, including financial projections, are estimates. The question is, Are they reasonable estimates?

Once these estimates are made, the buyer's DCF is calculated for each potential acquirer. The difference between this value and the seller's DCF should represent the appropriate range of value for the hospital. A comparison of this range for all likely acquirers should give you a reasonable basis for determining fair market value as well as a strategy for dealing with competing bidders. Without the buyer's DCF, you have only half the valuation range. But keep in mind that this is how buyers calculate what they will pay! Thus, unless the DCF analysis takes into account the available synergies for likely buyers, it will not replicate the market or reach the right estimate of fair market value. The result will virtually always be the significant undervaluation of the true worth of your hospital.

The second common methodology, the *comparable-companies analysis*, attempts to establish the value of the hospital being acquired (usually a single, stand-alone community hospital) by using the per share stock price of publicly traded hospital companies. In our view, using this method is like trying to establish the fair market value of the business of a street vendor selling hamburgers in your town by using the price of a share of McDonald's Corporation. We do not believe these are comparable companies at all, and the subjective judgments used to establish some sort of parity are easily challenged. Almost all the valuation experts we have discussed this method with, be they investment bankers or valuation consultants, view it as the least reliable of the methodologies. When seriously challenged, they often admit that it is really not used to establish value at all.

The third method commonly used, *similar-transaction analysis*, is the method that, in theory, most closely replicates the market. Using this methodology, experts attempt to find sales of similar stand-alone hospitals. Appropriate adjustments are then made for size, asset base, profitability, market anomalies, locale, and other relevant factors, and an estimate of value is then reached.

Although this method is theoretically closest to a market-based analysis, it does have some inherent shortcomings. The most important is that it is not the way buyers value hospitals. When you go to sell your house, the real estate agent often provides you with a list of sales of comparable properties in the neighborhood. You can use these past sales as an indication of value and establish your of-fering price consistent with them. In that instance, the similar-transaction method is extremely valuable. However, hospital buyers use a DCF analysis with their synergies calculated in. Because those synergies differ significantly depending on the location of other hos-pitals owned by that company and other factors, one can seriously question the ability of any valuation expert to make reliable adjust-ments to the price of one hospital so that it is "similar" to your hos-pital—yet such "adjustments" are the heart of this form of analysis.

Another problem with this method is that the data base on which it relies is weak. A great many transactions are made on a confidential basis, and so normally there are insufficient public transactions on which to base a reasonable conclusion, and, in ad-dition, the ones that are public may be too dated to be of much use in the rapidly changing hospital market. Therefore, the data base of a valuation expert using this method is inherently flawed.

Finally, there is a problem with the accuracy of the information in the public domain. When we review the "similar" sales provided by analysts, the numbers are often incorrect for transactions with which we are familiar.

Nonetheless, this type of analysis remains the most market-based of the three principal methods used and, properly done, is the one that provides the closest tie to actual market data.

Marketing Your Hospital

Once you have hired the appropriate experts, addressed manage-ment and expert conflicts of interest, and decided how to negotiate the deal, you are ready to begin the marketing process. The mar-ketplace will determine who the actual bidders will be, but you can influence the outcome to your advantage in significant ways by de-signing the marketing method to be used. A number of factors need to be considered.

Soliciting Interest by Buyers

It goes without saying that the more buyer interest you have for your hospital, the better off you will be. Accordingly, one of the principal tasks of the investment bankers will be to try to interest as many potential buyers as possible in order, first, to guarantee that you receive the highest price and, second, to insulate the board from potential criticism that it did not receive the highest price.

Getting the Bidding Started

Soliciting interest by buyers does not require formal bids. Investment-banking firms can and often do poll prospective buyers to determine their interest in a particular hospital. And, in any case, before you solicit formal bids, you should develop a request for proposals (RFP). The RFP serves multiple functions. It formalizes the nonprofit's description of what is being sold and lays out the format for bidding. Bidders can then submit bids that conform to the seller's demands. It also allows the seller to compare the bids received, knowing that they address the board's criteria as spelled out in the RFP.

In addition, the RFP contains a description of the assets being sold and other key terms that are important to the board. The extent to which working capital assets, such as accounts receivable, are included should be described, as well as any proposals for dealing with adjustments, provisions for assumption of liabilities by the buyer, and payment provisions (such as all cash versus notes or stock). The RFP is also the document in which you describe the terms of your offering to prospective buyers. Therefore, any special provisions you are intent on adding must be included, such as provisions for preserving mission statements or dealing with particular facilities or services. Because the RFP is the offering document, great care must taken in designing it and deciding precisely which assets and what terms will be included. It is the initial tool for generating buyer interest in your hospital, and good advice from your investment banker about how to make the offering attractive to buyers will be crucial.

One of the benefits of preparing the RFP is that it forces the selling nonprofit and its advisers to focus on the possible price impacts of various provisions in the sale terms. Selling any asset with restrictions on its use will affect the price a buyer is willing to pay. So insisting that the buyer adopt your mission statement or that it maintain certain facilities or services for the community, however laudable a goal, may lower the price you receive for the hospital. A lower price, in turn, reduces the financial strength of the surviving foundation and its ability to carry out a charitable program. If a board wishes to include such provisions in its RFP, it should, with the help of its advisers, evaluate the price impact of each restrictive provision to determine whether the provision is worth the price. The board's evaluation should be documented, and if it decides to include restrictive provisions, its reasoning should be documented as well.

Auction Sales: Optimizing the Possibility of Obtaining Fair Market Value

Once you have determined the universe of interested buyers, the next issue is how you deal with them. In our experience, auctions are the best method for securing the highest price. One example tells the story. In a sale of three hospitals owned by a nonprofit corporation in California, the seller conducted an auction in which several for-profit companies were the bidders. The initial valuation opinion provided by the nonprofit's expert for the three hospitals was $110 million. The opening bid in the auction was $112 million. Three weeks and four rounds of bidding later, the winning bid was $184 million—the free market does in fact work! The process of having three interested buyers compete in the fairest way possible resulted in an increase of $74 million above the initial valuation estimate, and all of that increase accrued to the surviving charitable foundation. It would be difficult to achieve similar gains without using the multiple-bidder (auction) process, which is one effective way to maximize price.

Your investment bankers are familiar with auction methods, so consult them about the variety of ways in which auctions can be conducted. Some examples will help you understand the possibilities. One seller conducted what it called a "double-blind" auction. With this method, the bidders were never told exactly what the other bids were or who the bidders were. After each round of bidding, the bidders were told what their rank was among the three bidding firms for that round. This forced each bidder to decide at every round of bidding how high it could go in the next round rather than how little it could bid over the next highest bidder. In this way, the seller was able to induce the bidders to put their best price on the table in each round. Another example is common in probate sales. It involves setting a minimum price for each round of bidding, normally a specified percentage above the highest bid in the last round. The bidders are told the highest bid in the previous round and are given the opportunity to continue in the auction only if they overbid that by a minimum percentage.

If the nonprofit is selling more than one hospital (or a variety of assets), it must consider whether to allow (or perhaps require) the bidders to bid for the assets separately or to purchase all the assets together. This is largely a strategic decision that the board needs to make in consultation with its investment bankers.

Single-Bidder Sales: "Shopping the Deal" and Protecting the Price

In many situations auctions are simply not feasible. What do you do if only one buyer expresses interest in your hospital or if, for strategic reasons, you believe it advantageous to target a single potential buyer? Although the law in virtually all states permits you to proceed without an auction, doing so exposes your board to substantial risks. Without a process that tests the entire market, you can never be sure that you received fair market value. And, more important, can you demonstrate that you did to your attorney general should he or she question the deal?

The best solution, if you can negotiate it, is to include a provision in your agreement stating that if another buyer surfaces—or if your attorney general requires it—the deal can be taken back to the market in a final attempt to solicit another bid. This solution normally requires a waiver of the "no-shop" clause in the letter of intent, a common provision that prohibits the seller from seeking other buyers after the letter of intent is signed.

These are the usual terms for a "back to the market" process:

- A guarantee that the initial deal remain binding during the "back to the market" period.

- A limited time frame. This should be the minimum time necessary for prospective new bidders to do their due diligence.

- A minimum overbid to ensure a meaningful increase in value. This process has costs and you need a significant overbid to make it worthwhile.

- A "breakup" fee. Often you will have to give the original bidder a monetary payment to reimburse it for its costs if an overbid comes in and is successful. Obviously, you will need to take this cost into account in establishing the minimum acceptable overbid.

Key Tip! You should use this tactic only if your buyer will guarantee its bid during the period when an additional bid is sought. Otherwise you risk losing the deal simply because of the possibility that a better deal is out there. We do not recommend taking this risk.

This type of provision allows the selling hospital to test the market for all potential buyers to see whether a higher bid is out there. If there is, the hospital has the right to secure that higher bid and force the original bidder to beat it. This procedure provides the hospital with an assurance that it has received the highest available price for its assets, and it protects the board members from both criticism and potential liability.

We have required this process twice in California, and both times the buyer guaranteed its price and terms during the re-market process. In the first instance, no additional buyers surfaced, and the original deal closed on time and as originally negotiated. In the second instance, an additional buyer did surface, and the eventual purchase price was increased by a net $20 million.

Choosing the "Best" Offer

One question often posed is, Can we consider factors other than price in determining what the "best" offer is? In our view, price will almost always be the determining factor in a straight cash sale. However, the board can, within the parameters of the business judgment rule, determine that other criteria are relevant as well. For example, the board may decide that continuing particular services or maintaining particular facilities (a burn unit or an ob-gyn department, for example) that might otherwise be shut down is so important to the community that continuing their operation should be made a condition of the transaction, even though this condition may discourage potential bidders or lower the sale price of the hospital. Other criteria might include the buyer's willingness to maintain the hospital's mission statement or a particular level of charity care for the community, the quality of the management of the buyer, the quality of other hospitals operated by the buyer, and the history of the buyer's relationships with its medical staff or employees. These criteria should be established before receiving bids. In this way, bids will be evaluated objectively and in accordance with the predetermined selection criteria.

In a 1996 sale of a multihospital system in California, the board not only had detailed selection criteria but also ranked the importance of the various criteria and assigned values ranging from 0 (low or negative satisfaction of criteria) to 10 (high satisfaction of criteria). This point system was used to evaluate the final bids from the three firms that participated in the auction. These were the criteria used:

- Bid price: measured as net to the charity at close

- Ability to close: perceived ability to complete the transaction with minimal price adjustments, as ascertained from language in contract offers, meetings with key bidders, and input from bankers

- Quality of organization: perceived quality of the bidders as ascertained from physician evaluations, reputation of bidders' other hospitals, and evaluations by senior management of the selling hospital

Interestingly, the firm selected came in second in the point system but offered a significantly higher price than the competing firms.

Documenting the Agreement

Once the bidding process is complete and a buyer has been chosen, the next step involves documenting the agreement of the parties to the transaction.

Letter of Intent

Usually, a letter of intent (LOI) is the first document created and signed. It sets forth the principal terms of the agreement, establishes a time frame for completion of definitive agreements (see below), and provides for confidentiality during that time. LOIs commonly include the no-shop clause discussed previously, which prevents the hospital from seeking other buyers during the time the final sale documents are being negotiated.

In addition to describing the major terms that the buyer and seller have agreed to, the LOI should also describe the major terms of the transaction that remain to be negotiated. Including these terms serves two purposes. First, it focuses the negotiators' attention on those areas that need to be resolved, thereby easing the way to final negotiations. Second, it signals to both parties whether they are sufficiently in agreement on the key issues to be able to reach a final agreement. The LOI can be either binding or nonbinding, although nonbinding is more common. The LOI should state expressly whether it is binding or nonbinding. With a nonbinding LOI the parties are not committed to either sell or buy the hospital until a definitive agreement acceptable to both is completed. They are bound only to negotiate in good faith for the period of time agreed to in the LOI. A nonbinding LOI creates only an agreement to attempt to agree or a moral obligation to continue negotiations. If you intend to have the LOI be binding, then you must be sure that you have negotiated all the terms that you need to be concerned about.

A good way to determine whether your LOI covers all the essential terms is to review another transaction between a nonprofit hospital and the buyer bidding on yours. That documentation will probably outline the types of issues that need to be thought through and agreed to before you conclude that you are ready to commit to a binding arrangement.

The signing of the LOI is often the trigger for publicly announcing a proposed transaction. Accordingly, it is a good idea to be certain that the basic terms not only are fair to the seller but also will not raise red flags with or substantial opposition from affected constituencies. If you can quell anticipated opposition in advance, you will greatly smooth the selling and the regulatory processes. If substantial opposition arises after a proposed transaction is publicly announced and if the opposition can point to problems with the proposal that the selling board did not anticipate, regulatory approval will certainly be more difficult, slower, and more expensive than it would otherwise be.

Definitive Agreement

The definitive agreement is the document that sets out the rights and obligations of the buyer and the seller with respect to the sale of the hospital. The process of negotiating the definitive agreement is crucial to the successful completion of a sale. Such documents are extraordinarily complex and require the advice of experienced financial advisers and transaction counsel on all sides. The key provisions will vary from deal to deal, although two important points common to all transactions require emphasis: the description of the assets and the conditions for closing.

An accurate and complete *description of the assets* being sold to the buyer and of those being retained by the seller is crucial. Often, buyers will express interest in purchasing assets related to your hospital, such as MSOs, but only after they have approved the financial condition after a period of due diligence. If they do not approve the condition for a particular asset, they will not be obligated to buy unless the definitive agreement imposes that obligation on them. In one case a buyer decided not to acquire an MSO that managed the practices of the doctors affiliated with the hospital; the selling charity was left holding an asset that was essentially valueless without the associated hospital, and it faced substantial liabilities associated with unwinding the business of the MSO. Obviously, if a buyer insists on and gets the right to reject certain assets during the due diligence period, the selling board needs to know what its exposure will be if the buyer exercises that option. And it needs to know that in advance of signing the definitive agreement.

We have found it quite helpful for the selling charity to have its financial advisers prepare a postclosing pro forma financial statement, which shows what the assets and liabilities of the charitable corporation are expected to be immediately after the transaction closes. If the board does not fully understand the financial risks contained in the terms of a definitive agreement, it may be unpleasantly surprised when the deal is complete and the amount received is less than anticipated. These risks can include both understated liabilities and overstated assets.

In one case a selling nonprofit board promised in its definitive agreement that there were no liabilities associated with an MSO being sold along with the hospital that had not been disclosed in the financial statements provided to the buyer. After the agreement was signed, several doctors participating in the MSO discovered substantial claims for uncollected receivables. As a result, the buyer, exercising rights under the warranties and representations provisions of the definitive agreement, demanded that the seller indemnify it for all costs of disposing of the doctors' claims. Such situations can lead to multi-million-dollar adjustments in the price actually received by the buyer.

Another risk arises from representations made with respect to the assets to be included in the sale price. It is not unusual for parties to agree at the time an LOI is signed to set the price on the assumption that the seller's level of working capital will be maintained as of a certain date. Similarly, parties frequently agree that the outstanding receivables will be fixed at a certain level and will be collectible. However, the time between signing an LOI and signing a definitive agreement can be lengthy. If substantial changes in working capital or the collectibility of receivables occurs, and the seller has agreed in the definitive agreement to the price provision of the LOI, the seller could face substantial downward adjustments in the amount it receives at close. If the amount received by the selling charity is considerably less than anticipated, it could affect the ability of the surviving charity to carry out planned activities.

Regulators will ascertain whether the selling board was negligent in failing to foresee such potential problems and deal appropriately with them during the definitive-agreement negotiating process, and if negligence by the board caused losses, the regulators will look to the board to recover the losses. Although directors' and officers' liability insurance may cover some or all of those losses, large deductibles can leave individual board members exposed to personal liability for the uninsured portion of the claims. And, in sale transactions, the losses can easily exceed the directors' and officers' coverage limits.

Key Tip! If there are contingencies in the deal that affect the price the buyer pays, the pro forma should spell out the range of possible results. Such a pro forma statement will help focus the selling board's attention on the possible risks that reside in the definitive agreement's terms before they are executed.

Another critical provision of the definitive agreement deals with *the conditions required to close*. This provision describes all the events that must happen before the seller is obligated to sell and the buyer to buy. If there are special conditions that you need to protect your interests, they must be in the definitive agreement. For example, it is not unusual for the parties to specify the required governmental approvals that must be secured before they are obligated to close the transaction. These can include approval by licensing authorities to transfer required licenses to the buyer, antitrust reviews, and if necessary under your state law, approval of the attorney general. In some cases uncertainty over whether specific uses of the funds by the surviving charity would be allowed by the attorney general have led to provisions in a definitive agreement requiring approval of the charitable-uses plan as a condition of the seller's obligation to close. Depending on when and how such approval is obtained under your state law, such a condition could be a serious negotiating obstacle.

The complexity of definitive agreements mandates that the selling board receive the advice of experienced professionals for all phases. Preagreement planning, negotiation, and post-agreement compliance are all difficult matters. To protect yourself from personal liability for mistakes, it is essential that you get the best advice you can, document that advice, and follow it.

Conclusion

The decision to sell your hospital is the most significant decision you will ever make as a trustee of charitable assets. It will affect your community, and it will affect you personally. Properly done, it can maximize the value of the hospital to the community, take advantage of favorable market forces, and provide substantial sums for charitable services to the public, the beneficiaries of your charity.

Improperly done, the sale of your hospital can cost your community substantial money, expose the directors to enormous personal financial liability, and seriously damage the reputations of both the hospital and its board of directors.

The best protection against these dangers is a market-based process. If you engage all potential buyers, obtain competitive bids, and consider them carefully, you will have essentially immunized your board of directors against charges that they obtained less than fair market value. Any other process, no matter how well done, will always leave questions about whether the best deal was obtained and will entail board exposure. Even in a nonauction process, however, these risks can be reduced. The advice we have provided is intended to help you to meet your legal responsibilities and avoid these pitfalls. These goals can be met through care, diligence, and selection of the right process.

5

Joint Ventures

The joint venture has become a popular and somewhat controversial form of conversion for nonprofit hospitals. In a joint venture, the selling nonprofit typically transfers its hospital to a new for-profit entity (usually a limited liability company), while the for-profit buyer normally contributes cash that is used to pay off the tax-exempt debt of the hospital. As a result, the two partners each own a percentage interest (based on the value of the assets each contributed) in the joint-venture entity. In most cases, the joint-venture entity is debt-free at the close of the transaction. The parties negotiate the terms of an operating agreement that dictates their rights to share power, management responsibility, and income from the venture.

The legal viability of this form of conversion has, however, come into question. In 1997, a trial court in Michigan ruled, at the request of the Michigan attorney general, that the 50/50 joint venture was illegal in that state because the assets of the joint venture were not dedicated exclusively to charitable purposes. Then, in early 1998, the Internal Revenue Service issued a decision (Revenue Ruling 98-15) that appeared to bar nonprofit tax-exempt corporations from engaging in virtually all forms of the joint venture currently in use. Again, the reason is that joint ventures are not entities whose assets are dedicated primarily to tax-exempt purposes. Nonprofits that participate in such ventures now do so at the risk of losing their tax-exempt status. Nonprofit hospitals that have already entered into such arrangements may be forced to unwind them.

Although it is likely that new forms of joint ventures will be developed by the for-profit sector to try to match the intricacies of the Internal Revenue Service ruling, the terms of that ruling will make such efforts difficult. The key requirements imposed by the IRS on the nonprofit partner are these:

- Governance: the majority of the governing board of the joint venture must be chosen by the nonprofit.

- Control: key decisions of the joint-venture board relating to the selection of management, distribution of earnings, changes in services, renewal or termination of management contracts, and capital and operating budgets must be subject to control by the nonprofit board majority (without the votes of the for-profit partner).

- Proportion: the nonprofit must receive a share of the joint venture equal in value to its contribution of assets.

- Purpose: the governing instruments of the joint venture must include an overriding charitable purpose and an express provision subordinating financial profit to the charitable purposes of the entity (in essence, creating a for-profit company with a charitable mission statement and subordinating the directors fiduciary duty to the financial success of the venture to the charitable mission).

In addition, the revenue ruling questions whether the joint venture can contract with the for-profit partner to provide management services or allow the for-profit partner to place its employees in key management positions. Each of these conditions creates a substantial impediment to traditional joint-venture models.

However, one or two new joint-venture models are designed to meet some, if not all, of the revenue-ruling standards; and we anticipate that additional models will be created. We do not expect the joint venture to disappear as a model, so you must be familiar with the key issues that will arise in joint-venture transactions.

Tip! Before considering any joint-venture proposal, board members should obtain a formal written opinion from both tax counsel and charitable-trust counsel that the proposed form of transaction complies with the law.

You should also keep in mind that, even where technically legal, joint ventures are difficult to negotiate in a way that protects the nonprofit's interests. Experience shows that the financial returns from joint-venture arrangements often do not meet the expectations of the nonprofit partner, and a failure to protect the charitable assets can end up exposing the board to significant risk of personal liability. So beware, this form of transaction carries a particularly high risk for the nonprofit partner; be sure the benefits are both achievable and worth that risk.

The joint venture's principal attraction is that it allows the nonprofit board of directors to remain engaged in the hospital's ongoing operations, although it is now a for-profit hospital. Often the board members have a strong attachment to the hospital after years of volunteering their time, effort, and money, and the joint-venture structure seems to them less an "abandonment" of the hospital than an outright sale of the institution to a for-profit chain.

Although it is possible to use this structure to maintain some level of board involvement in the hospital's ongoing operations and to safeguard programs important to the community, often the hoped-for benefits prove illusory. The nonprofit board finds that it has made significant financial concessions in return for "program assurances" that are unenforceable in the courts. And, needless to say, if your "program assurances" are not enforceable in court, they do not justify the monetary concessions.

Nonprofit boards of directors must, therefore, take extra care when considering the joint-venture structure. The legal and valuation issues are far more complicated than in an outright sale of assets. In addition, other critical issues arise regarding the terms of the joint operating agreement itself and the ability of the nonprofit to meet its charitable-trust obligations after the close of the transaction. These issues are further complicated by the existence of a continuing business relationship with the for-profit partner.

Keys to a Successful Joint-Venture Agreement

Negotiating a joint-venture agreement that satisfies the board's fiduciary obligations is never a simple task. There are, however, six basic rules for negotiating such an agreement that can help ensure that you meet your obligations. These rules will not guarantee a profit, but if the joint venture ends up being unsuccessful, complying with these rules will at least protect your charitable assets from undue losses and will preserve your ability to move those assets into other investments.

Rule 1. Do not invest all the nonprofit's assets in the joint venture. Diversify the nonprofit's investments. Following this rule will allow you to meet the capital needs of the joint venture without losing your veto powers or suffering unnecessary dilution (as explained below).

Rule 2. Insist on the right to appoint a majority of the governing board and to create an overriding charitable purpose that is reflected in the governing documents of the joint-venture entity. Following this rule will give you substantial control over your investment and the decisions that can affect it, and doing so is probably required by Revenue Ruling 98-15.

Rule 3. Insist on the right to veto major decisions that threaten profitability. Following this rule will help to ensure that you profit from your investment.

Rule 4. Minimize management's ability to dilute your ownership interest. Following this rule will protect your
appointing power, your veto powers, and your profit
participation.

Rule 5. Get a fair-market-value put (as explained below). If the
venture is not profitable, following this rule will let you
out of it without suffering large losses of your invested
capital.

Rule 6. Monitor joint-venture operations vigilantly to ensure that
you can exercise your powers under the agreement to protect your interests. This is the principal requirement of
the duty of due care.

The Typical Joint-Venture Model

The typical joint-venture proposal calls for the nonprofit to transfer its hospital(s) to a new for-profit company, formed as either a
limited liability company (LLC) or a limited liability partnership
(LLP). (See Figure 5.1.) The for-profit buyer puts in an agreed-upon
amount of cash, which is often sufficient to pay off the outstanding
tax-exempt debt of the hospital as well as provide operating capital
for the new for-profit venture. This cash contribution by the for-
profit partner can vary substantially and is a crucial part of the negotiation between the partners. The two parties then own the LLC
in agreed-upon percentages and negotiate an operating agreement
that governs their respective rights and duties in managing the joint
venture. Traditionally, the for-profit partner has the right to manage the day-to-day operations of the joint venture, and the two partners share control of the board of the new company. Sharing
control, however, does not necessarily mean that it is shared equally.
In our experience, the for-profit partner has always ended up being
the controlling partner in these joint ventures.

Figure 5.1. Simplified joint-venture model

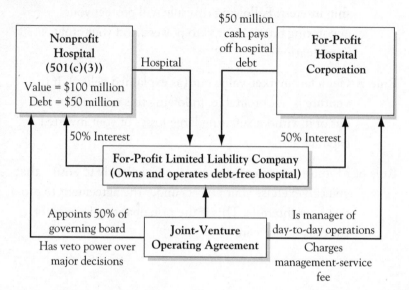

Advantages

The joint-venture structure, at least in theory, offers advantages to both the nonprofit seller and the for-profit buyer. For sellers, the joint-venture model combines the opportunity to secure skilled, for-profit managers and access to the public capital markets in a time of increasing financial pressures on hospitals. It can provide rights to an income stream from a greatly reduced or debt-free hospital operation. The joint-venture model also gives the nonprofit board shared control over certain major decisions concerning the hospital's future, thus providing it with some input into decisions concerning the community's access to medical services. In addition, the operating agreement generally permits the joint venture to bring in additional partners, typically managers and doctors; doing so allows the partners to align incentives to maximize profit opportunities in ways that are difficult for nonprofits to achieve.

However, these advantages come with a price tag, and the non-profit board must assure itself that the advantages are real and worth the price. A number of the methods used to bring in physician partners have been questioned by federal regulatory authorities. In addition, providing the for-profit partner with day-to-day management authority may create problems under Internal Revenue Service rules. Proposals regarding either of these items should be thoroughly reviewed by legal counsel prior to including them in any agreement.

Risks

The nonprofit faces the following serious risks when entering into a joint venture with a for-profit partner, especially if the for-profit partner will manage the venture:

- The value of the nonprofit's assets going into the venture not being equal to the value of the joint-venture interest received

- Operating-agreement terms that cause below-market returns on the nonprofit's investment

- Dilution of the nonprofit's ownership in the venture with corresponding loss of control

- Profiteering by the for-profit partner through management fees and service contracts between the joint venture and the for-profit or its subsidiaries

- Lack of access to the capital invested in the joint venture.

Joint-venture interests in privately held entities are difficult to value and to sell, assuming you are even allowed to sell under the terms of the agreement. The value in the open market of the interest of the noncontrolling partner is always significantly discounted because of a lack of control and lack of marketability. Thus, the nonprofit partner, who will almost always be the noncontrolling partner within the joint venture (regardless of the number of board seats it controls), faces a large loss in the value of the assets it puts into the venture. Two carefully negotiated provisions in the joint-venture agreements can help protect against this loss of value: (1) a guaranteed market for the nonprofit's joint-venture interest and (2) legally binding assurances that the nonprofit partner will receive fair market value for the assets it put into the venture, with no discounts for lack of marketability or lack of control.

The amount of attention that needs to be paid to the terms of the operating agreement cannot be overstated. Unless careful attention is paid to those terms, the nonprofit may find itself earning far less from its joint-venture investment than it could have earned from other readily available investments. Low earnings can have numerous causes. For example, if the for-profit managing partner has the power to reinvest the joint-venture earnings in capital improvements to the joint venture instead of distributing the earnings as profits to the partners, it has every incentive to do that because it is likely to want to buy out the nonprofit's interest in the hospital ultimately.

Another major risk the nonprofit runs by becoming a "captive" noncontrolling partner is not being able to leave the venture without suffering a substantial loss of its capital investment while being faced with dilution of its interest; this dilution in turn may threaten the shared control of the venture—the basic motivation for using this structure in the first place. Dilution of the nonprofit's interest in the venture can happen in several ways. For example, in a 50/50 joint venture the nonprofit seller often retains few or no liquid assets at the close because all or most of the cash put into the transaction by both parties is used to pay off tax-exempt bonds and to provide working capital. The nonprofit is, therefore, unable to meet demands for additional funds ("capital calls") that the managing partner has the right to make to improve the facility. Failure to meet capital calls, under most agreements, results in a reduction of the nonprofit partner's proportional share of the venture. Your charity's ability to participate in decision making (normally called shared governance) is likely tied to retaining a certain minimum ownership share; multiple unmet capital calls can reduce your interest below the minimum level required to keep the charity's voting rights and powers in the joint venture.

Another source of dilution is the addition of new partners, usually managers or affiliated doctors. Again, unless protections are built into the agreement, dilution can result in loss of the nonprofit's ability to control major operating decisions, thus wiping out one of the principal attractions of the joint venture in the first place. The joint-venture model will have allowed the buyer to acquire control over a presumably desirable hospital operation (and perhaps even entry into a new market) at half the cost of an outright purchase!

Another major risk the joint venture poses for the nonprofit partner is that the for-profit partner can use its power as the venture manager to direct a disproportionate share of the income stream to itself. This diversion can be accomplished in a variety of ways such as charging excessive management fees or negotiating "sweetheart" vendor contracts with wholly-owned subsidiaries of the for-profit partner. The result is a below-market income stream for the nonprofit and a further reduction in the value of its investment.

The final risk with the joint-venture structure that must be avoided is lack of access to the capital the nonprofit has invested in the joint-venture partnership. You must insist on the right to sell your interest in the joint venture to your partner at fair market value without discounts. Such provisions, known as "put" or "option-to-sell" provisions, give the board assurance that its interest in the joint venture will be saleable at fair market value whenever it wishes to sell for any reason. Without such a provision, there is unlikely to be any market for your interest, or if there is, its value will be discounted significantly. No nonprofit should even consider a joint venture without a put.

A variety of put agreements are possible. The terms of such a provision that need to be considered include (1) the length of time the put will be in effect, (2) the method for determining the put price, (3) the conditions under which the nonprofit will be allowed to exercise the put, (4) the method of resolving any disputes over exercise of the put, and (5) whether the put will be exercised with respect to some or all of the nonprofit's interest in the joint venture and who decides. These terms are discussed in detail later in the chapter.

In sum, as a nonprofit trustee, you must ask these questions about a joint venture:

- Do the governance provisions of the agreement really protect you?

- Can the for-profit partner dilute your joint-venture share?

- What will your rate of return on the joint-venture interest be and will you get it?

- Can you carry out a charitable program?

- Can you get out of the joint venture without the loss of charitable assets?

Policy Analysis

The nonprofit's usual motive for entering into a joint-venture arrangement with a for-profit entity is to retain some board control over the hospital while, at the same time, improving its financial outlook through a strategic affiliation with a financially stronger for-profit partner. This decision is usually made after the nonprofit suffers losses or determines that it is likely to begin to incur losses that threaten its continued viability. The nonprofit board must address a variety of issues to determine whether a joint venture is the best approach to resolving the concerns that motivated consideration of conversion in the first place. If other motives, such as the continuation of basic medical services for the community, motivated the board's decision to seek a joint-venture arrangement, it must ensure that the agreements meet those goals. Simple assurances that your prospective partner will maintain a trauma center or retain all your employees are worthless if they are not enforceable. If such provisions are important to your assessment of the deal, make sure the they become binding contractual agreements.

Investment Analysis

The commitment of all or a substantial portion of a nonprofit's assets to a joint venture is a significant investment decision, and among the many questions nonprofit hospital directors must ask themselves is whether the proposed transaction is a prudent investment. That question, in turn, raises issues of diversification of risk, access to capital, and marketability of assets. A nonprofit board will face three major decisions:

- How much of the nonprofit's assets will be put into the joint venture?

- Is the value of the joint-venture interest the nonprofit will receive equal to the value of the hospital assets it will put into the venture?

- Are the risks of making the joint-venture investment appropriate in light of other investments the nonprofit might make with the same assets?

Failure to understand any of these issues is a failure to comply with the nonprofit board's duty of due care.

What Percentage of Your Assets Will You Invest?

The first, and most fundamental, decision facing a nonprofit board considering a joint venture is how much of the nonprofit's assets to place at risk. Although there are no set rules, there is an analytical model to help boards address the issue. Assuming the hospital is the nonprofit's sole significant asset, the 50/50 joint-venture model typically requires the nonprofit to contribute almost 100 percent of its assets to the joint venture. However, other configurations allow for greater diversification. For example, a 90/10 agreement, with the nonprofit owning 10 percent and the for-profit partner owning 90 percent, yields an investment ratio by the nonprofit in the joint venture of 20 percent of its total invested assets. To use an example from the simplified joint-venture model in Figure 5.1, the nonprofit would have to invest $10 million of its $50 million in net assets to purchase a 10 percent interest in the debt-free joint venture.

Similarly, an 80/20 joint venture yields an investment ratio by the nonprofit in the joint venture of 40 percent of its total assets. Again, using the simplified model of Figure 5.1, the nonprofit would have to spend $20 million out of its net assets of $50 million to purchase a 20 percent interest in the joint venture, yielding an investment ratio of 40 percent. Finally, a 75/25 joint venture yields an investment ratio of 50 percent. The nonprofit in the simplified model would have to spend $25 million, or half its assets, to buy a 25 percent interest in the joint venture.

As these examples highlight, as the percentage of the joint venture that the nonprofit partner wants to buy increases, so does the percentage of its assets required to make the purchase and, more important, so does the risk from lack of diversification. This risk in turn increases the board members' exposure for any losses that might result from the joint-venture investment.

Will Your Returns Equal the Value of the Assets You Invested?

In a joint venture, valuation of assets is a particularly complicated task. To begin, the nonprofit must know the value of the assets it is putting into the joint venture. If the board conducted an auction in which several bidders participated, you can be confident that the market process established the fair market value of the assets. If the nonprofit did not conduct an auction or if only one potential partner was interested, it will be more difficult to know whether any particular valuation for the hospital assets equals fair market value. This is a significant problem because, in most states, the board is prohibited from transferring any assets to a for-profit entity at less than fair market value. (See, for example, California Corporations Code, § 5917.)

To further complicate the valuation issue, the nonprofit must assure itself that the value of joint-venture interest it gets in return for its hospital equals or exceeds the value of the hospital and other assets contributed to the joint venture. This is the most difficult and the most important issue in a joint-venture transaction.

A number of factors can reduce the value the market will place on that interest:

- Loss of management control

- Risk of dilution of the charity's interest

- Inability to ensure profit distributions

- Inability to sell the charity's interest

If you give up too much control over management of the joint venture to your partner, the market will treat your interest as noncontrolling and discount its value significantly. We have received opinions from experts suggesting that the market would discount such a noncontrolling interest by as much as 45 percent. In such a case, the investment is almost certainly ill-advised, and pursuing it may create personal liability on the part of the board members.

To illustrate, using the example from Figure 5.1, assume your nonprofit hospital enters into a 50/50 joint venture with a for-profit hospital chain by transferring your hospital to an LLC, and the for-profit is to be the managing member of the LLC. The net result is that both partners have a net investment of $50 million in the venture and a 50 percent interest in the LLC. If you have not negotiated an operating agreement that fully protects your charity, the interest you receive could be discounted in the market by $22.5 million ($50 million × .45). That is also the measure of your personal exposure for failure to exercise due care.

Could You Do Better Elsewhere?

Before you commit your nonprofit to the difficult and expensive process of finding a joint-venture partner and putting together an appropriate deal, you should analyze whether the likely returns on this investment are at least as good as those available from other prudent investments. The fiduciary duty of due care requires that you make a reasoned determination of your likely return on investment and decide that the return is both worth the risk and as good as you could reasonably expect from alternative prudent investment opportunities. You will not satisfy the duty of due care if you make an investment without a reasonable idea of the return it will generate.

Although there are no assurances for your rate of return, at a minimum your advisers should be able to provide you with a pro forma for the first year of operations of the joint venture. A pro forma is a written estimate of the projected income from operations, usually based on the historical operations of the hospital, adjusted in this context by the expected improvement in management that the new partner will bring and the fact that the debt of the joint-venture entity will, in most instances, be less than it currently is. Using assumptions about the efficiencies expected to be achieved by the new management, the pro forma subtracts projected costs of operations to arrive at projected profits. Such a pro forma will enable the nonprofit board to compare the projected return on investment in the joint venture with other possible investments.

A pro forma should also be prepared for the surviving charity. This pro forma should show the financial picture of the charity at the close and again at the end of the first year of operations. This is another tool for the nonprofit board to use in assessing the wisdom of the joint venture proposal. It will allow the board to determine whether it will have sufficient funds to conduct a charitable program after it enters into the joint venture.

The creation of these two pro formas will force you to work through major provisions of the proposed joint-venture agreement to understand how they work. This exercise, in turn, will allow your board to determine whether its interests are adequately protected by the proposal. Ultimately, you want to know what the estimated rate of return will be on your joint-venture investment before you sign the agreement.

Process

If you have decided to pursue the joint venture, the board must develop a process designed to ensure that it satisfies its fiduciary obligations as it addresses the unique problems of the joint-venture format. These are the three most critical issues to address:

- Be sure the board understands the joint-venture structure.

- Develop a procedure that ensures that the corporation receives fair market value for its assets.

- Negotiate transaction documents that protect the nonprofit's interests.

In order to accomplish these goals, it is imperative that the board retain qualified, independent professionals to assist in evaluating all aspects of a proposed joint venture. And because each issue, in turn, raises complicated questions that may require varying types of expertise, the board should be prepared to hire a variety of specialists in different fields.

Understand the Issues

The best advice about hiring experts is to do it as early as possible. Because critical decisions often have to be made at the beginning of the process, the earlier the board secures appropriate advice, the better its decision making will be, and the community or regulators will be less likely to challenge choices supported by sound decision making.

First, you need to address the tax-law questions raised by Revenue Ruling 98-15. Before you do anything else, retain tax counsel to advise you what form of joint ventures can be considered without jeopardizing your tax-exempt status. We believe that this ruling makes it difficult to devise a joint venture that makes good business sense, so be particularly careful in this area.

Second, you need to address valuation issues. The board should get advice from investment bankers, valuation consultants, or appraisers with experience in handling hospital transactions, and it should do so before it authorizes any discussions with potential buyers. Waiting until after the price has been discussed with potential buyers (or, worse, after an agreement has been reached) will invariably result in a valuation skewed to justify the price already discussed or agreed to. Such "backward-looking" valuations are far less credible to regulators than valuations made at the start.

Most valuation firms will be able to advise the board about the value of the assets it is putting into the joint venture. However, this is not the key valuation issue. As we explained earlier, the key issue is valuing the joint-venture interest that the board is to receive in exchange for its hospital. This is an extremely complex issue, and few firms have the expertise or the experience to assist the board. Thus, it is critical for the board to explore the qualifications of potential advisers to assist with this issue, which is unique to the joint-venture model.

Get Fair Market Value

Marketing your hospital is complicated by the fact that the board has decided to seek a joint-venture arrangement. Not all potential buyers will be as interested in a joint venture as they would be in some other structure, whether a sale, a lease, or some sort of management arrangement. This fact necessarily has an impact on the value that will be received for the assets. Different potential partners may have different ideas concerning the types of joint operating provisions they are willing to include in a joint-venture agreement. Such differences will affect both the value of the LLC or LLP interest and the ability of the nonprofit to protect its interests once the arrangement is finalized. This is true as well for the buyout, or put, arrangements that are critical to protecting your ability to secure fair market value for your joint-venture interest.

It is, therefore, crucial that the board get the advice of experienced firms in developing a marketing plan that allows it to do the following:

- Accurately compare competing proposals

- Determine the risks of competing proposals

- Determine which proposals meet the objectives that led to the board's considering a joint-venture model in the first place

More simply said, the board needs to use an evaluation process that ensures that it is comparing apples to apples when it considers different proposals.

Make Sure the Deal Documents Protect You

Finally, when it comes to the most difficult process of hammering out the actual transaction documents, the board will need the help of experienced advisers and attorneys. Neither directors of hospitals nor their in-house counsel have the experience to negotiate this sale. And you must recognize that the firms that acquire hospitals—those on the other side of the table—have a great deal of experience and have developed expertise in negotiating these types of transactions. The nonprofit board is at a substantial disadvantage from the start in negotiations with sophisticated buyers. The best way for the board to protect its interests when considering such a transaction is to secure the best advice it can from experts with experience in these types of business arrangements. Do so at the outset of negotiations.

Protecting Yourself and Your Hospital

To protect yourself and your hospital during the process of finding your joint-venture partner, be sure to do the following:

- Understand the limits of your expert's ability to advise.

- Let the market work for you.

- Pursue your values, not someone else's.

- Evaluate comparable proposals.

- Be wary of using selection criteria other than price.

Understand the Limitations of Your Expert(s)

We recommend strongly that a nonprofit board hire the experts it needs to understand and grapple with the difficult issues involved in negotiating a joint-venture agreement. However, we add the caveat that the board must understand the limitations of the experts it chooses as it evaluates their advice. Although the board is entitled, from a fiduciary point of view, to rely on the advice it receives from experts in making important decisions (see Chapter One), the board's reliance on that advice must be reasonable. Remember, the ultimate responsibility for any decision lies with the board, not with the experts it has retained.

In dealing with experts retained to advise the board, every board member (or at least every member of the special committee of the board appointed to handle the transaction) must be sufficiently conversant with the issues confronting the board to be able to ask appropriate questions about the advice received. In this way each board member—not a select two or three—meets his or her fiduciary duties. In addition, the board must take steps to eliminate, or at least account for, any conflicts of interest on the part of its advisers that might color their advice and adversely affect the nonprofit's interest in the transaction.

A few examples will highlight these points. On valuation issues, a board might reasonably hire an experienced investment-banking firm to advise it both on the initial valuation of its assets and on the plan for marketing the hospital to particular joint-venture partners. Although the investment-banking firm may advise the board about the value of its hospital, that opinion is not a substitute for testing the market by attempting to secure at least several comparable bids for the hospital. The investment-banking firm's opinion may be colored by a number of factors, including its relations with for-profit acquirers and its desire to obtain a commission.

If the board fully appreciates these limitations on the advice it gets, it can take steps to minimize, if not eliminate, any adverse effects from such potential conflicts. For example, hiring one firm to provide the board with strategic-planning advice, including the initial valuation, and a second to conduct the marketing and sale of the hospital would eliminate any tendency on the part of the merger and acquisition firm to underprice the assets for a quick sale. In fact, it would provide the board with a check on the initial firm's work product. The method of compensating the firm or firms hired can also be used to reduce the risk of conflicts. For example, paying a fixed fee for the initial valuation eliminates any concern that the firm will be influenced by the outcome of its work. Conversely, contingent percentage fees may provide incentives to the firm hired to market and sell the hospital to maximize the price received so as to maximize the fee.

The board should consider all aspects of the proposed arrangements with experts and document its process of considering and selecting its experts, as well as its reasons for compensating those experts with the chosen mechanism. Careful documentation of the board's decision-making process and of the reasons for its decisions is an important way of satisfying, in part, the board's duty of due care.

The most critical area in which experts prove useful is negotiating the terms of the joint-venture operating agreement. This document determines everything that happens in the future in your joint venture. The board may feel that its own management is best able to evaluate the adequacy of the proposed operating agreement. But how many joint-venture operating agreements has your management team negotiated? How many joint ventures have they previously been involved with and how did they work out in practice? If a deal turns out badly, these are the questions your state attorney general is likely to ask you, and these questions are going to be asked to determine whether you breached your duty of due care in assigning this responsibility to management.

Let the Market Work for You

It goes without saying that the board's most basic obligation in entering into a joint venture is to secure fair market value for the charitable assets it is putting into the venture. Any failure on this score not only damages the charity but exposes the board members to personal liability for the difference in value between the assets put into the venture and the assets received in exchange. The surest way to achieve fair market value is to expose the transaction to the widest possible market. If the board can create multiple competitive bids for its desired transaction and then takes the best deal, by definition the board has secured fair market value.

The difficult problems arise when, for any number of reasons, it is not possible to expose the hospital to a large number of potential partners. The board's investment advisers may find out in the process of contacting potential partners that only one or two firms are interested in the hospital. Alternatively, the board may have placed constraints on the adviser in regard to the qualifications of potential partners, and these constraints may eliminate some or perhaps many potential partners from being considered. When these situations arise, the board's duty of due care requires that it take all appropriate steps to match as closely as possible the results that would be achieved by a fair and open marketing process.

Pursue Your Values, Not Someone Else's

Whether you believe that there will be many potential partners bidding for your hospital, a few, or only one, the board must develop an appropriate procedure for meeting the goals it has set for the transaction and maximizing the value the nonprofit ultimately receives. What that procedure should be will depend in large measure on the number of potential partners who are genuinely interested in the hospital.

If you have several parties interested in your hospital, some variation of the auction method will virtually guarantee that you maximize the value received. Make sure that you have not placed unnecessary constraints on bidders that may adversely affect the price you receive. For example, your board may feel that the maintenance of particular facilities at the hospital is a desirable goal. If so, make sure you document your consideration of whether there are less costly ways of providing that service to the community than requiring the joint venture to provide it. You do not want to put yourself in the unfortunate position of having paid the highest price for a service because you chose to force the job on your joint venture rather than testing the market for alternative suppliers.

Evaluate Comparable Proposals

If you are fortunate enough to have several firms bidding for the right to engage in a joint venture with you, you must ensure that you have a reasonable basis for choosing one proposal over another. Insist that your investment banker or other advisers develop an RFP that forces the buyers to bid on the same transaction. If you do not, you cannot be sure that you are comparing equivalent proposals. You should also develop a list of the criteria that you will use to evaluate the bids. If access to public capital markets is important to you, put that factor on your list and let the bidders know. If maintenance of professional relations with medical staff is important, put that on the list and make sure your RFP requires the bidders to provide information so you can compare firms in this regard. In summary, when the bidding is over, you want to be comparing apples to apples and oranges to oranges. Anything less will create confusion on the part of the bidders, stress for your board, and fodder for opponents of your transaction.

Price is the area where similarity of proposals will be most important. If one bidder is guaranteeing a certain income stream for some period of time and the others are not, it is difficult to compare the real prices being offered by all. If one firm is offering all the management services necessary to conduct the business of the joint venture while others insist on the right to contract separately for various management services, that fact must be accounted for in comparing price. The nonprofit board simply should not put itself in the position of making impossible comparisons between varying offers.

To illustrate this issue, we once reviewed a transaction in which the selling nonprofit received joint-venture proposals from three different firms. The proposals were different from one another in major respects. The valuations of the proposals also varied widely. In fact, the range of difference was nearly $200 million in the view of some experts, thereby opening the nonprofit up to criticism no matter what it did. This type of problem can be avoided by using the right process from the start and having clear criteria for selecting the joint-venture partner.

Be Wary About Using Selection Criteria Other Than Price

Nonprice factors may be important to the nonprofit board. After all, by choosing this format, you are deciding to go into business with the winning bidder. So, of course, you can consider nonprice factors. Nonprice factors that might be important to you include (1) the quality of the management skills and systems of the bidders,

(2) the willingness of the bidders to maintain certain services, and (3) the reputation of the bidders. But, as with all other decisions you make in this process, your discretion is limited by your duty of due care. Can you choose a firm with perceived excellence in management systems over firms with lesser skills in that arena at a cost of several million dollars or even tens of millions? You can, but you had better be able to demonstrate that the return will be better over time, and you must document those reasons. There are no bright-line rules in this area. But if you intend to select a bidder that has offered lower prices than the others, you need to be able to justify that choice. If the price differences are small, justifying the choice may be less difficult. As the price differences get larger, so will the difficulty of justifying your selection.

Structuring the Transaction

Assuming you have made a decision to proceed with the joint venture, the process of negotiating the transaction agreements typically begins with an LOI. This document sets out the bare-bones agreement that you expect to negotiate and provides for a period of exclusive negotiations. Next, the contribution and sale agreement describes the assets being put into the venture by both partners, the liabilities to be assumed, and the assets and liabilities that are excluded. It also sets out the principal terms of the financial arrangements for structuring the joint venture, such as the price to be paid for the assets going into the venture, the percentage to be owned by each partner, and the conditions to be met before each partner is irrevocably committed to the deal. The third, and most important, document to be negotiated is the joint-venture operating agreement. This document defines each partner's rights and obligations in conducting the business of the joint venture. Finally, if there is to be a buyout agreement, or put, it may be included in the joint operating agreement or placed in a separate agreement. All four documents are discussed below.

Letter of Intent

The major purpose of the LOI is to describe the basic transaction the parties have agreed to negotiate. The LOI is a necessary part of the process of reaching agreement and presents several important opportunities to the parties. The critical features of the LOI are (1) memorializing the basic agreements the parties have reached, (2) defining the issues that still must be resolved, (3) committing the parties to further negotiations, and (4) deciding whether the LOI is to be considered a binding contract and, if not, what events will allow either party to terminate discussions. Properly done, the LOI will facilitate the negotiation of the definitive agreements necessary to complete a transaction.

Negotiating the LOI provides an opportunity for the parties to test their willingness and ability to agree on difficult issues. The parties also get their first taste of working together, an opportunity that should not be overlooked; the parties are, after all, planning a long-term working relationship. Finally, drafting the LOI tells both sides about the quality of their respective team's negotiating abilities.

Certain issues must be addressed in the LOI:

- Structure of the deal, price, and payment terms

- Exclusivity, confidentiality, and timing of negotiations

- The agreements and conditions that need to be completed

- Termination rights and whether the LOI is binding or not

First, the parties should describe the essential terms of the proposed deal, the assets to be included, and the price. If the joint venture is to be a 50/50 partnership in an LLC, now is the time to say so. Second, the parties typically agree to negotiate exclusively with each other for some period of time and to keep the negotiations confidential. Third, the parties define the issues that need to be completed by negotiation. And, finally, the parties must decide whether the LOI is intended to be a binding commitment, and, if not, what events will allow either party to terminate the negotiations.

Contribution and Sale Agreement

The contribution and sale agreement (CSA) is the final contract between the parties. You will need the advice of experienced transaction lawyers to negotiate and document the CSA. Because every deal is unique, we cannot describe all the details that need to be addressed in your CSA, but certain provisions are common to all CSAs and essential for each:

- Description of parties, assets, price, time, and conditions for close
- Representations and warranties of each party to the other
- Preclosing obligations of each party
- Conditions precedent to each party's obligation to close
- Routine provisions for indemnification, noncompetition
- Close or termination of agreement

First, you must set forth the essential terms of the agreement in a way sufficient enough to make it a binding contract. These include the parties, the included and excluded assets, the consideration being paid by each party, the time for closing, and any procedures the parties must complete to accomplish the transaction.

Second, the CSA should contain all representations and warranties the parties will be required to make to the other. Third, all preclosing obligations of both parties must be set out. Fourth, all conditions precedent to each party's obligation to close should be defined. Fifth, all mechanics of the transaction such as indemnification, due diligence, noncompetition agreements, and provisions regarding medical records should be set out clearly. Finally, the CSA must provide for either closing or terminating the obligations of the parties.

Operating Agreement

The crucial difference between a sale and a joint venture is that upon the signing of the joint-venture agreement the parties plan to conduct a business together. And the "heart and soul" of the joint venture—the document that defines the business relationship—is the joint-venture operating agreement. We have never seen a joint venture in which the for-profit joint venturer was not the managing partner, with day-to-day management responsibilities. It is thus essential that the nonprofit partner ensure that the terms of the operating agreement protect its rights. Without adequate provisions in the operating agreement, the nonprofit loses substantially, both in its ability to guarantee community benefits and in its ability to protect its share of the joint venture's cash flow.

Under Revenue Ruling 98-15, joint ventures with the for-profit partner having broad management authority are likely to be impermissible for charitable corporations. As a result, we expect that the for-profit industry will revise its models in an attempt to comply with the new rules. No matter what form of partnership is proposed, it will almost inevitably be the joint venture operating agreement that defines the respective rights of the parties. In order to protect your charity's rights, do not lose sight of this fact.

These are the key provisions of the operating agreement that the nonprofit partner must have:

- The right to appoint a majority of the joint-venture board members

- The right to veto major decisions of the managing partner

- The right to force profit distributions

- The right to prevent dilution of interest by admitting new partners and making capital calls

- The right to control management fees

- The right to force the managing partner to buy the nonprofit's interest at fair market value on demand

As in any other entity, *the right to appoint the governing board* is critical to controlling the business of the joint venture. Under Internal Revenue Service rules, the nonprofit will be required to have the right to appoint the majority of the joint venture's governing board as long as it remains in the partnership. You must therefore be careful to insure that there are no provisions in the agreement that would eliminate your right to appoint 50 percent plus one of the board members. If that right is not granted, you will be compelled to sell your interest or risk losing your exempt status. Pay close attention to provisions that could dilute this right!

The joint-venture agreements we have seen have provided that the nonprofit's right to appoint board members is eliminated if its ownership share drops below a specific percentage. The powers of the governing board and the conditions under which the nonprofit can lose those powers are obviously pivotal to the charity's ability to ensure that it gets what it wants from the joint-venture arrangement.

The governing board is often given power over a wide range of transactions, although these vary from agreement to agreement. In effect, as long as the governing board retains power over key decisions and the nonprofit maintains its requisite percentage of control (whether defined as ownership percentage or voting percentage), it maintains a veto over the major decisions. The range of issues that can be covered by these governance provisions depends on the parties; these issues may include (1) selecting the joint venture's chief executive officer, (2) selling major assets of the joint venture, (3) making capital expenditures over agreed-upon amounts, (4) borrowing more than agreed upon amounts, (5) deciding for how much and when cash distributions should be made, (6) approving contracts between the joint venture and the managing partner of the joint venture or its affiliates, (7) dissolving the joint venture, (8) entering into business combinations with other entities, (9) amending any of the agreements governing the joint venture, or (10) deciding which medical programs will be offered by the hospitals owned by the joint venture.

Another important protection the nonprofit partner should have in the operating agreement is the *right to veto key decisions* of the managing partner. Because the nonprofit typically enters the joint venture for a variety of reasons, including increased access to capital, managerial efficiency, and economies of scale, it tends to focus on reserving powers over community-benefit issues. This may be an appropriate allocation of responsibilities under the joint-venture agreement. But the nonprofit board needs to think about its veto powers as the essential tool for fulfilling its fiduciary duty to protect the charitable assets it is trading for the joint-venture interest. If the nonprofit cannot protect the value of its joint-venture interest with the veto powers it negotiates into the operating agreement, it cannot satisfy its fiduciary duty of due care.

The next question the board must address is, Are these provisions enforceable and do we have the will to enforce them? If the answer is no, you will have given up something of value for nothing, to the detriment of the charitable interest. Remember, no one else is going to enforce these provisions for you. So you must ensure that the veto powers are legally binding in the agreement and clear enough to be understood and enforced by the courts.

The major decisions that the nonprofit should be concerned with protecting by the veto power include those that are essential to ensure that it receives an adequate return from the cash flow of the joint venture. The nonprofit should insist, at least, on veto powers over capital expenditures, annual budgeting, borrowing money, determining cash distributions, entering into service agreements with the managing partner or its affiliates, and any other provision of the operating agreement that affects the joint venture's profitability.

The provisions for *profit allocation and cash distribution* are among the most complicated provisions of the operating agreement. They are also the most important if the nonprofit expects to earn a return from the joint venture. Accordingly, special care must be taken to ensure that the nonprofit board understands how they work.

The most important feature of the profit-allocation provisions of the operating agreement is that allocations are tied to the partners' ownership percentage, just as you would expect. Thus, the dilution problems we discussed above will have a direct impact not only on the nonprofit's ability to control the manager's running of the joint venture but also on the nonprofit's earnings from operations.

The second most important feature is that profits are usually defined as the joint venture's "taxable income." All joint-venture costs of operations will therefore reduce profits for allocation purposes. To the extent that the for-profit manager can direct expense payments to itself or its affiliates, it reduces the profits available for the nonprofit, while increasing cash flow to itself.

Besides the profit-allocation provisions of the agreement, the board needs to understand the cash-distribution provisions. These provisions determine when the partners in the joint venture will receive distributions of cash from operations. Typically, these provisions permit either the manager, with approval from the governing board, or the governing board itself to determine whether excess cash (over the needs of the company) is available for distribution.

Remember that approval of the board is generally tied directly to the voting percentage of the members. Thus, the ability of the nonprofit to preserve control over cash distributions is linked to whatever protections are built into the shared-governance provisions of your agreement. If you maintain veto powers down to low levels of ownership, then you keep control. If you lose veto powers in direct proportion to your level of ownership, then the dilution-causing provisions (admitting new partners and capital calls) are critical to your ability to control cash distributions. If you lose control of the cash distributions, you lose the ability to maintain your income stream from the joint venture. If a large percentage of the charity's assets have been devoted to the joint venture and it cannot easily get out of the joint venture, the loss of control over the income stream could mean the elimination of charitable programs.

It should be clear by now that one of the most critical issues confronting a nonprofit considering a joint venture is the need to *protect against the effects of dilution* of its ownership interest. Under the current Internal Revenue Service rules, not allowing dilution is critical to retaining your tax-exempt status. Dilution can be caused either by adding new partners or by being faced with capital calls you cannot or will not meet; we will discuss both here.

Joint-venture operating agreements can provide for admission of affiliated doctors and managers as partners in the joint venture. Typically, the right to admit new partners is subject to the approval of the governing board, while the managing partner is given the power to set the price the new partners must pay for their interests. The admission of new partners can dilute your ownership percentage and your voting rights. You need to protect against both.

You need to understand the dilution risks that admitting new partners poses in any joint-venture agreement you are thinking about. First, and most important, do not allow this provision to give the manager unfettered authority to admit additional members to the joint venture. If you do, you will be authorizing dilution of your ownership and voting interests, which threatens your continued ability to legally participate in the partnership. If there is conflict among the partners in the future, the additional partners are likely to align themselves with the for-profit manager rather than the nonprofit for voting purposes. Admitting new members will change the balance of power in decision making. Thus, the nonprofit must understand those provisions of the operating agreement where voting percentages are important and protect its rights.

Second, the admission of new members will dilute the nonprofit's ownership and voting percentage and thus bring it closer to the threshold for losing representation on the governing board. So it is equally important for nonprofits to understand fully all the provisions of the agreement that can reduce its voting percentage. If you do not understand these provisions, you cannot assess the wisdom of agreeing to the addition of new members.

You should not give the managing partner complete discretion in pricing the sale of units to new members. Instead, either reserve pricing authority in the governing board, so you retain control, or require the manager to sell new partnership interests at fair market value. If you do not, the manager will be able to buy the loyalty of the new partners by offering them rights to buy in at a discount. We have seen partnership admission provisions that require that the consideration "be based on fair market value," but that is not the same as requiring that they be sold for fair market value. A sale of units to management at 50 percent of fair market value is "based" on fair market value. But such a sale price will certainly result in admitting management personnel likely to vote with the manager. Discounted sales of units to new members will lower the investment value of the nonprofit's ownership of units because its share of the distribution will go down by the percentage of new units sold, and it will not receive fair market value for such units because of the discount offered by the manager.

The other major source of dilution of a nonprofit's interest in a joint venture is the obligation to meet capital calls made by the managing partner. A capital call is simply a demand that the partners contribute more money to the partnership. But these contributions are not loans, they are investments in the business. So, when you meet the capital calls, you put that money at risk.

Two types of capital calls are common in the joint-venture agreements we have reviewed. First, some agreements allow the managing partner to make capital calls to pay for significant additions to the plant of the hospital (often called "major capital expenditures") that have been approved by the governing board. Second, some agreements allow the managing partner to make additional capital calls whenever it "reasonably believes" that more funds are needed to meet the operating expenses of the joint venture. Typically, the operating agreements require the managing partner to make the capital contributions required to meet the triggering expense initially and then to call on the other partners to make their pro rata contributions. The other partners are given a choice of meeting the capital call or suffering a loss of either their ownership percentage, their voting percentage, or both, to the extent they choose not to meet the capital call. Both types of capital-call provisions pose serious threats to the ability of the nonprofit partner to maintain its ownership or voting percentages. These threats, if realized, can damage the nonprofit's ability to protect its investment. Accordingly, nonprofit boards considering such ventures must take steps to minimize the risk of such provisions or provide a mechanism to escape their impact should they occur.

Each of these types of capital call needs to be fully understood by the board. The first type allows the managing partner of the joint venture to make capital calls to pay for major capital expenditures that have been approved by the governing board. The fact that approval of the board is required for major capital expenditures provides some protection against dilution of the nonprofit's interest because the nonprofit can simply refuse to approve particular major capital expenditures. However, if the nonprofit has approved major capital expenditures for any particular year, this provision gives complete discretion to the manager to determine whether the joint venture "needs" additional funds to pay for the expenditures. Exercise of that discretion by the manager can lead to reduction of the nonprofit's share of ownership of the venture if it is unable or unwilling to meet the required capital call. If the nonprofit has contributed virtually all its assets to the joint venture (the 50/50 venture), the nonprofit could be exposed immediately to loss of ownership share by such provisions.

Two types of protection should be considered to avoid this threat. Reducing the nonprofit's share of the initial capital of the joint venture will leave the nonprofit in a better cash position and enable it to meet capital calls if it needs to. However, meeting capital calls from the charity's funds obviously reduces the ability of the nonprofit to carry out its charitable mission. So it is important for the nonprofit to build other protections against dilution into the operating agreement.

The second protection the nonprofit should consider is making the right to make additional capital calls one of the major decisions requiring approval by the governing board. This requirement is somewhat cumbersome because it requires a board meeting every time the managing partner thinks that additional capital is needed. However, it does give the nonprofit an added level of protection against dilution and permits the nonprofit to insist on other methods of raising funds, such as loans, that do not dilute its interest in the venture.

Capital-call provisions that give the manager the right to decide when additional capital is "reasonably necessary" for operating expenses pose a great dilution threat to the nonprofit for two reasons. First, they give the manager discretion to make capital calls for expenditures that may not have been approved by the governing board. Second, conferring discretion on the manager to determine when additional funds are needed to carry out the business of the joint venture is an open invitation to the manager to make additional capital calls that threaten the nonprofit's ownership or voting percentages. As in the case of the call for major capital expenditures, this provision typically requires the manager to make the expenditure in the first place and then seek pro rata contributions from the other partners. If the other partners choose not to or are unable to meet the call, they suffer reduction of their ownership percentage and their voting percentage.

It is crucial for the nonprofit to be aware of and account for these threats to its ownership and control rights before it commits itself to the transaction. Again, the nonprofit can gain a significant degree of protection simply by committing a smaller percentage of its total assets to the joint venture and by securing a strong put, thereby guaranteeing an exit right at fair market value.

A significant threat to the nonprofit's ability to get earnings from the joint venture is the *manager's compensation*, often referred to as the management-services fee (MSF). The MSF is usually calculated as a percentage of the "net revenue" of the joint venture, usually 1 or 2 percent. However, net revenue is defined as the joint venture's gross revenues less contractual adjustments, bad debt, charity care, and administrative discounts. Because this calculation does not include the cost of operations, such as employees, plant, and overhead, the manager is taking its fees off the top!

In the agreements we have reviewed, the manager is expressly authorized to contract with its affiliates for the provision of management services, in addition to those services covered by the MSF. Expenses incurred for such additional services are also included in the costs of operations. Thus, the manager is earning substantial proportions of the joint venture's revenue stream before any provision is made for the nonprofit to share in that revenue. If profit margins are relatively thin, a not-uncommon situation for hospitals, the calculation of management fees based on gross revenues exaggerates the impact on the profits available to the other partners.

Consider, for example, a hospital that earns gross revenues of $100 million with an operating margin of 5 percent, making the profit available for distribution $5 million. A 2 percent management fee based on gross revenues would mean an MSF of $2 million, or 40 percent of the available profits of the joint venture. In this example, the manager would earn its $2 million MSF, plus its 50 percent share of the balance, assuming no new partners have been added, or an additional $1.5 million dollars. So the manager earns a total of $3.5 million compared with the nonprofit's $1.5 million in this simplified example. Stated differently, the manager earns 70 percent of the net proceeds from operations. And these figures do not even account for the possibility that the manager will employ its affiliates for additional services. Obviously, the nonprofit wants to carefully consider entering into an agreement skewed so heavily in favor of the for-profit partner.

The nonprofit also needs to understand what the MSF pays for and what it does not pay for. In the agreements we have reviewed, the parties define carefully the management obligations of the manager. Often, those definitions are set out in a separate schedule of the operating agreement. That schedule is usually designed to limit the management services that the for-profit is obligated to provide in exchange for its MSF. We have seen three types of management services defined in operating agreements. First, the schedule defines those services the manager is required to perform for its MSF. Second, the schedule defines those additional services the manager will provide to the joint venture at additional expense at its discretion. Third, the schedule defines yet more services the joint venture is authorized to request and for which the manager will be paid additional fees. In the agreements we have reviewed, the for-profit partner attempts to give itself the discretion to choose which services it will provide to the joint venture and at what price. All these additional expenses for management services detract from the funds available for distribution as profits to the partners.

If the differences between these categories are not understood by the nonprofit, it will lose earnings as the manager simply shifts the available cash from operations into purchasing more services from its affiliates. In effect, the nonprofit pays twice for the manager's services: once with the MSF and again with reduced profits caused by the expense of so-called additional management services.

The "Put"

The nonprofit board must also *protect its ability to gain access to its investment* in the joint venture. A joint-venture interest that cannot be sold or that can be sold only at substantial discounts because of lack of control is an interest that you should not own. If you agree to a joint venture without guaranteeing both access to your investment and access without a substantial minority or lack-of-marketability discount, you will suffer a huge loss in the value of your joint-venture interest the day you sign the agreement.

Therefore, it is not, in our opinion, ever prudent to enter into a joint venture that does not have a buyout provision, called a "put." The put is a guarantee that the for-profit partner will buy out the nonprofit partner's interest under agreed-upon conditions. In essence, the put creates a market for the sale of the joint-venture interest where one would not exist otherwise. To be prudent, the put should last the life of the agreement and should require the for-profit partner to pay fair market value (without discounts for lack of marketability or lack of control) when the put is exercised. This type of provision ensures that the trustees will always be able to get out of the deal and to exit at fair market value if they decide that is prudent. Anything less exposes the trustees to liability for the difference between the fair market value of the assets it put into the joint venture and the value received should the board decide (or be forced) to sell.

The put is your master insurance policy. If the venture is not as profitable as hoped or relations with the manager break down for other reasons or the nonprofit simply wants to convert its investment to cash, the put gives the nonprofit partner the ability to sell its interest. Without a put the nonprofit almost certainly will not have a market for its interest because few investors would be willing to buy a minority interest in a hospital operation controlled by someone else.

Properly structured, the put guarantees the nonprofit both access to its capital and protection for the value of its asset. We recommend that the nonprofit insist on a put that requires the for-profit partner to buy out its interest based on the fair market value of the hospital operation as a whole; this is the provision that protects value. The actual price would be determined by applying the nonprofit's ownership percentage at the time the put is exercised to the fair market value of the whole enterprise of the joint venture. This method protects the nonprofit from loss of value due to minority discounts that the market might apply in valuing interests that lack control over the business enterprise.

We also recommend that the put last for the life of the operating agreement; this is the provision that protects access to capital. We believe that such a provision is preferable to fixed-term puts. If a put is negotiated for a limited term, as the deadline approaches it will become clear that the nonprofit must exercise the put. If the term expires without its exercising the put, the nonprofit's interest in the joint venture will not be marketable or will be marketable only at a greatly discounted value. At that point, the nonprofit will never again be guaranteed access to its investment at fair market value, regardless of changes that may occur in the value of that investment. We do not believe a nonprofit board can put itself in that position with respect to a significant percentage of its assets and comply with its duty of due care.

The put can apply to all of the nonprofit's interest in the joint venture or to agreed-upon percentages of its interest, which can be sold in stages. We have seen put provisions that require the nonprofit to sell 100 percent of its interest if it exercises the put. Such a provision has the advantage of ensuring that the nonprofit does not sell a portion of its interest and thereby fall below the operating-agreement thresholds for loss of its veto power. But such a provision is not required. A nonprofit could negotiate the right to sell its interest in blocks of 10 or 20 percent of its interest (probably expressed in terms of the number of joint-venture units). If such a put is considered, the nonprofit needs to pay careful attention to the effect of partial sales on its veto power and its voting rights under the terms of the operating agreement.

Finally, the method of setting the purchase price for the assets if the put is exercised needs to be carefully considered. Because it is unlikely that the joint-venture interest can be sold under market conditions, the parties need either to agree on a purchase price or to resort to some sort of appraisal mechanism to set the price. Whatever method is chosen, the essential feature, in our view, is the requirement that the nonprofit not suffer a minority discount in selling its interest. The reason is simple. If the nonprofit were to sell its hospital under open-market conditions, it would not suffer a minority discount. The decision to consider a joint venture should not leave the nonprofit in a worse position than a sale. If it does, the board faces personal exposure for the loss in value.

Conclusion

Internal Revenue Service rules call into question the viability of the joint venture as a conversion format. Even assuming that such questions can be overcome by changes in the joint-venture format, joint ventures pose issues that are unique and difficult for nonprofit boards. Valuation issues are especially difficult because of the need to value both the assets being put into the joint venture and the interest being received. Operating and management issues are crucial to protecting the value of the nonprofit's investment and its ability to receive income from the venture. Protecting against dilution of the nonprofit's interest is essential. And most important, the need to guarantee access to the nonprofit's capital investment with a put cannot be overstated.

While these issues are difficult, they are not impossible. Because the joint venture offers attractive business features to both the nonprofit and for-profit partners, we expect new models to be developed that will satisfy the Internal Revenue Service rules and the demands of trust law. A nonprofit board considering a joint venture must ensure that the model it chooses complies with both. A failure on either count will expose the board to unnecessary risk of personal liability.

6

Legal Protections for Directors and Trustees—and the Consequences for Failing to Use Them

Nonprofit hospitals depend on community leaders to bring their talents, business skills, and judgment to the boards of these critical community facilities. Serving as a nonprofit trustee is one of the highest forms of meeting the call to civic duty. Accordingly, the law provides certain basic protections against personal liability for decision making by directors and trustees of nonprofit hospitals. The law also provides serious consequences for actions that fall outside these protections. The purpose of the law regarding director and trustee liability is not to dissuade civic-minded persons from serving as directors of nonprofit organizations. Nor is it to punish directors for making incorrect business decisions as they try their best to manage these enterprises. To the contrary, the laws in all states are designed to encourage community leaders to participate in the nonprofit sector and to bring their business acumen and creativity to this sector. At the same time, the law recognizes the importance of safeguarding charitable assets from waste, mismanagement, diversion, or worse. The goal of the regulatory mechanisms established by most states in this area is to create a system that meets both goals.

Charitable-trust law tries to reconcile these goals by providing a series of protections, some procedural, some substantive, so directors can avoid personal liability for decisions that go awry. These are the protections and "safe harbors" provided:

- Business judgment rule

- Careful conduct rule

- Delegating responsibility

- Directors' and officers' liability insurance

- Indemnity

As a counterweight, significant legal penalties are imposed on directors who violate the law and fall outside the legal protections and "safe harbors" provided. These are the penalties that can be imposed:

- Breach-of-trust lawsuit with possible personal liability

- Removal as a director

- Internal Revenue Service intermediate sanctions

The bottom line is that directors who act in good faith, in a properly designed decision-making system, and without seeking personal enrichment at the expense of their charity should never face any significant risk of personal liability.

Legal Protections

The law provides two types of protections for directors to help them avoid personal liability for decisions that, through no fault of their own, go wrong. One type consists of legal doctrines that are designed to provide protection through process guidelines. These include the business judgment rule we discussed previously (see Chapter One) as well as the right to delegate responsibility for due diligence activities. The second type are tools that can be utilized to protect directors from financial risk. These include directors' and officers' liability insurance (D&O coverage) and indemnification.

Properly utilized, these measures can immunize directors from personal financial loss resulting from any liability they incur for decisions they make.

Business Judgment and Careful Conduct Rules

The business judgment and careful conduct rules provide the standards of conduct that regulators and the courts use to evaluate decisions made by nonprofit directors. Both these legal doctrines are intended to protect directors from liability exposure for making decisions. These rules are process-driven and can, therefore, be satisfied completely with a properly designed decision-making system.

However, in some circumstances, these rules can create exposure to personal liability. Our experience has shown that when these protections break down, the failure is invariably either in the area of "good faith" or in the area of "reasonable inquiry." Good faith often means the lack of a conflict of interest. If any member of your board of directors has a material financial interest in the transaction you are undertaking, and this includes your chief executive officer if he or she sits on the board, then your board is conflicted and does not meet the good-faith test. Therefore, your actions are likely to be judged under the more stringent test applied to self-dealing transactions, and failure to recognize this conflict in advance virtually guarantees that you will violate the law. The solution is clear: require your attorneys and managers to make full disclosure of any financial benefits to be received by any board member or officer, and get it in writing. This procedure will give the board the information it needs to determine the applicable fiduciary standard that must be met. There is no excuse for not demanding this information, and there is no excuse for your counsel and management to fail to provide it. If you ask for this information and do not receive it, red lights should start flashing.

The other area that can expose board members to personal liability is that of "reasonable inquiry." This doctrine requires board members to a make a reasonable inquiry into all facts pertinent to a decision the board intends to make. However, frequently, senior management or controlling cliques on boards of directors withhold relevant information from the full board, provide inadequate explanations and allow insufficient time for the full board to review proposals, or ask boards of directors to rubber-stamp management decisions. Each of these practices is an invitation to disaster—and to personal liability.

When a competent regulatory agency conducts its inquiry into a hospital sale, it will quickly identify the problem areas in the deal, whether they involve self-dealing, valuation defects, or charitable-uses problems. That regulatory agency will want to know why the board failed to identify and resolve these problems. The answer "We just did not know" is tantamount to an admission of negligence. It is your responsibility as a board member to know. So make sure you have the necessary information before you vote on any deal. It is not a difficult task. Keep in mind that you are required to make a conscious and informed decision. Ask the questions that need to be answered so that you fully understand the transaction and are able to determine whether it is in the best interests of the charitable corporation. Be sure that the answers to your questions are put in writing, and have those materials incorporated into the board minutes. Finally, make sure you know the right questions to ask. If you are unsure, ask your board to retain experts in the appropriate fields to explain the transaction and target the proper areas of inquiry.

These are simple and effective ways to ensure that you meet the standards of the business judgment rule and the careful conduct rule. Following these simple steps is the only way to obtain the protections these rules are designed to give you.

Always demand from your attorneys and your management the following:

- Complete disclosure of all financial benefits related to the transaction that are to be received by officers, senior managers, or directors

- A complete analysis of all trust restrictions that govern the charitable assets being sold or joint ventured—this requirement applies to both restricted endowment funds and to general corporate assets

- A complete description of all efforts made to sell, joint venture, or otherwise convert the hospital, including the RFP sent to prospective partners and summaries of all responses received

- A summary of the financial or other considerations that motivated senior management and the board to explore conversion in the first place

Obtain this information in writing and sufficiently in advance of the board vote so that you have time to review and digest it. Courts are likely to question the reasonableness of decisions of this magnitude made without adequate time to reach an informed decision.

If you feel that you have not received adequate information or advice after requesting it, demand that you be provided with independent counsel. Remember, corporate counsel are generally retained by management and their loyalties lie there. If you have requested from corporate counsel information that you believe you need to reach an informed decision and they have refused to get it to you, your corporate counsel is thereafter conflicted, and you should force the issue. It is the only way for you to protect yourself.

In the end, there is one rule that you need to follow religiously: do not vote for any proposal that you do not understand or that you do not believe is in the best interests of the charitable corporation. The decision to convert your nonprofit hospital is, without question, the single most important decision that you will ever make as a board member. You know this; the regulators know this; and the courts know this. The enforcement agencies and the courts will expect you to conduct the level of inquiry appropriate for a decision of this magnitude. And although the business judgment rule will protect you from a decision made after reasonable inquiry and in good faith—even one that turns out badly—it will not protect you from a decision made without such an inquiry. It also will not protect you in situations where conflicts of interest exist or where you did not understand the deal and make a reasoned decision on the merits.

If the deal is in the best interest of the charitable corporation, those advocating it should be able to explain it and justify it. If they cannot, there is probably a reason. Unless you are convinced, do not give them your vote. And never respond to pressure for a unanimous vote. A desire for unanimity is not a factor that regulators or courts will weigh favorably in determining whether you complied with your fiduciary duties.

Delegation, Reliance, and Other Safe Harbors

The law in most states permits you to delegate responsibility for due diligence to corporate officers, committees of the board, and outside experts and consultants. (For a full discussion, see Appendix B.) Most states also allow you to rely on those to whom you delegate that responsibility. This is an exceptionally valuable tool for avoiding personal liability, but it works only when you use it properly. Relying on the advice you receive from those to whom you have delegated responsibility for recommending decisions affords you substantial protection but does not give you carte blanche. Your delegation of responsibility and your reliance on the advice you receive must be reasonably exercised, and that is not terribly difficult to do properly.

We suggest a few simple rules. First, delegate responsibility to individuals who have skill and background in the area involved. Second, make sure that those to whom you delegate are not conflicted by an actual or potential financial relationship with the acquirer. Third, give those to whom responsibility is delegated adequate time and resources to do the job properly. Fourth, require those doing the due diligence to provide a written report to the board well in advance of a vote. Be sure the report addresses the key issues that were assigned and that are to be decided, and obtain an unequivocal recommendation for a course of action. Fifth, discuss the report at the board meeting and ask the other board members and your counsel whether they are aware of information or facts that would contradict the factual assertions or recommendations being provided. Do not go forward until those matters are fully resolved. And, finally, be sure your board minutes fully reflect all these steps. If you follow these rules, it is almost certain that your delegation and reliance will meet the requisite legal standards.

One final point should be made regarding the rules for legal protection. Regulators and state legislators are becoming increasingly sensitive to the inherent conflicts of interest that senior management brings to conversion transactions. Nonprofit board members understandably rely on their senior managers as these are the individuals responsible for the day-to-day operations of the hospital. However, in a hospital sale or joint venture, these individuals often have a significant conflict. The hospital is likely to be faced with competing choices that will translate into different employment opportunities or challenges for senior management. Where one of the options is a for-profit conversion, senior managers will, in all likelihood, hope to remain in their present jobs after the transaction. A takeover by a for-profit chain often brings the expectation of increased compensation, including bonuses and stock options. Senior managers may, therefore, be proponents of the conversion alternative if they perceive it to be in their financial self-interest. No individual can realistically be expected to disregard these pressures.

In California, the state legislature has recognized this problem and provided an interesting solution that includes simple rules and a safe harbor for directors who follow them. Senate Bill 413 (Peace), enacted in 1997, provides that directors of a converting nonprofit hospital may obtain input, information, and guidance from senior management. However, directors may not rely substantially on that information unless those managers have signed affidavits pledging that they will not work for the for-profit acquirer in the future. If the managers decline to sign that affidavit (and we expect that most will), the directors may still rely on the managers' input but only if they have hired an independent consultant to vet that information—in effect, providing a second opinion that is unbiased and accurate. Directors working under this law have no excuse for failing to protect themselves by following these procedures.

Other states have provided different rules to guard against conflicts of interest among senior management. In addition, Revenue Ruling 98-15 effectively prohibits nonprofit management from getting jobs with the new for-profit owner in a joint-venture transaction.

Protecting against management conflicts is especially important when senior management has been the force driving the decision to convert. Often, management's financial projections are used to convince the board that conversion is necessary for survival; usually management recommendations that a specific type of conversion is best-suited to continuing hospital operations dictates the form of conversion; management often negotiates the deal, in terms of both financial consideration and mission statements; and management likely selects the experts and counsel who guide the board through the approval process. If management is conflicted, all these decisions are suspect. Independent counsel or experts, selected by and reporting directly to the board, provide an important check on the process and should give the board of directors comfort that they have reached the right decision.

Directors' and Officers' Liability Insurance

Directors often ask whether they can protect themselves from personal liability even when they have made a serious error that constitutes a breach of trust. The answer is yes, and the method is to have your hospital buy directors' and officers' (D&O) liability insurance. D&O liability policies pay for directors' legal costs of defense and liability under certain circumstances, just as your car insurance pays for any legal costs and personal liability you may have for causing an accident. Many state nonprofit-corporations statutes specifically allow for such insurance to alleviate any legal question about whether its purchase is proper. (See, for example, California Corporations Code, § 5238(i).) A corporation can buy insurance policies to cover the corporation and its officers, directors, and employees. No one, in fact, should sit on a nonprofit hospital board without it.

D&O policies principally cover negligence with respect to either the duty of due care or the duty of obedience to purpose. These policies generally do *not* cover violations of the duty of loyalty, such as self-dealing or private inurement. In fact, some statutes, including California's, expressly prohibit coverage for violations of the duty of loyalty. In California, a review of standard insurance-policy language will reveal an exclusion for any act that is intended to benefit an officer, director, or employee personally. Typical policies read as follows: "The insurer shall not be liable to make any payment for loss in connection with any claim or claims made against the Directors or Officers or Trustees arising out of, or based upon or attributable to the gaining in fact of any personal profit or advantage to which they were not legally entitled." It is important to know what is covered by your policy, and reading it after the fact is not going to give you much guidance.

Most D&O policies are "wasting" policies; the costs of defending a case are deducted from the total amount of coverage, and so you may be personally exposed to some portion of any liability. Therefore, you should make sure that your charity has purchased sufficient coverage to pay for both the reasonable costs of defense and potential liability. It is also important to know whether your policy requires the insurance company to advance legal costs to defend a suit. The policy may not provide for payments until a settlement or judgment is entered. This requirement is normally covered under the policy's "duty to defend" clause. This language is usually fairly clear and reads something like this: "insurer agrees to defend and indemnify" (defense costs covered and advanced), or "the insurer does not, under this policy, assume any duty to defend" (defense costs not advanced). Check your policy. If it does not include a duty to defend, it is likely you or your charitable corporation will have to advance defense costs, which can be large.

In conversion cases, the key fact to keep in mind is that if you are going to engage in a self-dealing transaction with the acquirer, you are probably without coverage. For example, if one of the doctors serving on your board owns a lab affiliated with the hospital and that lab is being purchased by the buyer of the hospital, the director is engaging in self-dealing. Even if the self-dealing is fully disclosed to the board, unless you follow the steps required by your state law to secure regulatory approval of the self-dealing, you could face exposure to liability if a court later finds that the price paid for the lab was too high. And if that transaction is challenged by a regulatory agency, your personal finances will be put at risk regardless of the size of your D&O policy because most D&O policies exclude coverage for self-dealing.

It is also crucial to remember that not all D&O policies are created equal. Some exclude intentional acts; others do not. Some advance legal fees; others do not. Some exclude violations of a statute; others do not. Therefore, you should instruct your management to work with your hospital's insurance agent to obtain the best coverage available to meet your needs. You should also instruct your counsel to review the policy language before you buy to make sure it provides the right kind of coverage.

Finally, you should know that almost all D&O policies are "claims made" policies: the coverage you buy for the current year does *not* necessarily cover acts committed this year. It covers claims made against you this year. If you engage in a transaction in 1998, but that transaction is not challenged by the state attorney general until 2001, the insurance will provide you with no coverage at all. You will have to renew that coverage every year until the statute of limitations runs out on any possible claims, or you will not be fully protected.

This is important stuff. Make sure that you have adequate insurance, both in amount and breadth of coverage. Your financial security depends on it. Without insurance coverage, in a breach-of-trust lawsuit, the regulatory agency is going to look to your personal assets to make the charity whole.

Indemnification

Another method for protecting directors against personal liability is to include indemnification provisions in the articles of incorporation or bylaws of the charitable corporation. Simply put, these provisions permit the organization to pay judgments, settlements, or legal expenses incurred by a director charged with wrongdoing.

Most states that have enacted laws dealing with nonprofit corporations have authorized indemnification of directors, officers, and employees. (See California Corporations Code, § 5238; Connecticut General Statutes, 33-454(a); Illinois Revenue Statutes, ch. 32, para. 108.75; Louisiana Revised Statutes, 12:227; Montana Code Annotated, 35-2-411; Texas Corporations and Associations Code Annotated, 1396-2.22A.) These laws can set the allowable limits for indemnifying directors and trustees. The statutes may be "exclusive," providing that a corporation may never grant greater protection to its directors and trustees than that authorized by the statute, but permitting lesser protection. Or they may be "permissive," allowing broader indemnity. So you should check with your attorney to make sure that your corporation has authorized the maximum level of protection permitted under your state's law. These provisions are found in the articles of incorporation or bylaws and normally state that the corporation is "authorized to indemnify its directors to the full extent permitted by law" or some similar language. If your articles or bylaws do not contain this broad grant of authority, you should amend them to broaden their scope.

The law with respect to indemnification of directors is relatively uniform among the states. There are five key issues you need to consider:

- When is indemnification permitted?

- Who can approve the decision to indemnify me?

- Is indemnification mandatory or permissive?

- Will the indemnity include the cost of defense and any liability, and are there any limits?

- Are there acts the corporation may not indemnify me for?

If you know the answers to these questions, you can decide whether the level of protection that is available is sufficient. We discuss each of these issues here.

As a *general rule*, a charitable corporation may indemnify its directors for any acts done in good faith and with a reasonable belief that the acts were in the best interests of the charitable corporation. This should sound familiar! It is the same standard required to invoke the business judgment rule. You might ask, What good does this provision do then? If you satisfy the business judgment standard, you probably could not be held liable in any event. However, in a number of situations the ability to utilize the indemnification provisions in the articles does, in fact, provide a substantial benefit to a director accused of wrongdoing; foremost among those benefits is coverage in situations where there is a substantial risk that the D&O carrier will deny coverage and refuse to defend you.

Insurance carriers, not infrequently, raise objections to either paying a settlement or judgment or advancing defense costs. On occasion, they have excellent reasons for doing so; for example, the insured may have made misstatements in the policy application or may have performed acts expressly excluded under the policy, such as acts constituting a criminal offense. Although most D&O policies exclude coverage for criminal acts, most state indemnification statutes permit indemnity for criminal conduct provided that the person involved had no reasonable cause to believe the conduct was illegal. (See, for example, Colorado Law, § 7-129-102(1)(C).)

Also, you may choose not to buy a D&O policy that provides for defense costs. If you do, you may find yourself incurring enormously expensive legal fees to defend yourself. Virtually all state indemnity statutes provide for the advancement of defense costs pending a determination of liability. Having such costs covered can significantly contribute to your financial and mental well-being when litigation runs for years.

Most states have alternative methods for *approving indemnification requests*. The board of directors can usually authorize indemnification by a majority vote of those present at a meeting with a quorum present, counting toward the quorum only those directors who are not parties to the proceeding in which indemnity is being sought. If a quorum cannot be obtained, the board can designate a committee of disinterested members (usually two or more) to make the decision. Where such designation is not possible, state law often permits the determination to be made by independent legal counsel selected by a majority vote of the full board. In situations where there is a corporate member, that member is often authorized to make the decision. And, finally, most statutes provide for a court of competent jurisdiction to authorize indemnification.

Directors often ask, "Do I have an absolute right to be indemnified, or can my board say no?" The answer is that it depends on the circumstances. *Most state statutes contain both discretionary and mandatory provisions, with most situations covered at the board's discretion.* Thus, even if you meet the requisite standard, the organization is not required to indemnify you. It is not hard to tell these provisions apart. The discretionary sections say that the corporation "may" indemnify you, and the mandatory sections say the corporation "shall" indemnify you.

When does each type apply? Mandatory indemnification applies only where the director prevailed in defense of an action for wrongdoing. In some states, the law provides a different, and more generous, rule for outside directors. Those states require organizations to advance an outside director's expenses provided the director provides a written affirmation that he or she meets the standards for indemnification and provides an undertaking to reimburse the corporation should it be ultimately determined that the director did not meet the requisite legal standard.

The key point, however, is that lawsuits of the kind we have been discussing are often filed well after the events in question occurred. If the board membership has changed and the current members did not support the transaction or do not look favorably on those who approved it, they have the legal right to refuse your request for indemnification. Only if you prevail in court on the merits will you be entitled to indemnification.

Most states permit your corporation to indemnify you for damages and legal fees, and there are no arbitrary limits on the amount of the indemnity. This is one area in which indemnity provisions are more generous than insurance policies. All insurance policies have a specific limit on liability, and as we mentioned previously, costs of defense come out of that limit. Consequently, if you underinsure, you may find that you have covered your defense costs but have no coverage remaining to meet a damage verdict. This is a serious problem when a board is large and most, if not all, of the board members are named as defendants. If those board members have differing interests and require separate counsel, the costs of defense can escalate quickly. In California, it is unusual for charities to maintain coverage of less than a million dollars. In the case of hospitals, we often see coverage in the $10–15 million range.

Most states have special rules dealing with advances of funds to pay for defense costs. Even those that prohibit loans to directors usually permit advances to defray defense costs. Generally, directors seeking such advances are required to provide written undertakings to repay the amounts advanced should it ultimately be determined that they are not entitled to indemnification. However, statutes often authorize such an advance on an unsecured basis and without reference to the directors' ability to repay the advance.

Indemnification is particularly important where there is a problem with D&O coverage. Under most policies, the carrier picks up the defense costs automatically. However, if the obligation to defend is contested by your insurance carrier, indemnification by your corporation may be the only source other than your bank account for paying huge legal bills.

What cannot be indemnified? is probably the most important question. The law prohibits indemnification for certain types of acts as a matter of public policy. A general list of acts for which you are on your own is fairly easy to make. The law prohibits you from being indemnified for acts that justify punitive damages, fines, or penalties. These acts include fraud, willful misconduct, and, in many states including California, self-dealing or other acts of personal profiteering. Because these actions and penalties are also generally not included in your D&O policy you are wholly without protection for them: forewarned is forearmed.

Legal Consequences

The tools to protect officers, directors, and trustees from personal liability in their management of nonprofit corporations do not always work. What happens if these protections are not utilized or are not available as defenses for a particular action that your board has taken? What are the consequences of violating the law in this area?

Officers, directors, and trustees face three different kinds of legal actions when they violate the rules in handling charitable assets. First, and by far the most serious, is criminal prosecution. This sanction applies to the most egregious violations—generally the theft or embezzlement of charitable funds. These cases are normally prosecuted by the local district attorney's office. They almost always involve the use of charitable funds for the defendant's personal benefit. They are generally not board-approved and are often accompanied by concealment or falsification of records. They can result in prison terms, fines, and orders of restitution.

Because neither of us is a criminal lawyer and because these cases, although well publicized, tend to be rare, we will not discuss them in detail. Suffice it to say that such prosecutions do serious damage to the reputations and finances of both the individuals and the organizations involved. Judges and juries do not sympathize with individuals who abuse a position of trust to steal money from charitable organizations and from the poor and needy who depend on such organizations. And although state indemnification statutes often contain enabling language permitting the indemnification of directors in criminal cases, we have yet to see a such a situation. Attorneys general look with significant, and aggressive, disfavor on using charitable funds to indemnify officers or directors from the expense of criminal conduct, particularly when the victim is the charity itself. Simply put, this is one road you do not want to go down.

The vast bulk of enforcement cases do not, however, involve the criminal justice system. Rather, they fall into one of two other categories: charitable-trust civil-enforcement actions, usually brought by state attorneys general, or tax-law actions brought by the Internal Revenue Service.

Charitable-Trust Civil Actions

The primary enforcement tool for preventing breaches of trust and remedying those that do occur is a civil-enforcement action filed by a state attorney general. As we have discussed, state attorneys general have both common law and statutory jurisdiction to remedy breaches of trusts. They represent the public beneficiaries of charitable trusts under a doctrine known as *parens patriae*.

The most common method of exercising this jurisdiction is through a civil action filed against the officers and directors personally or against the charitable corporation or both. Although the range of potential causes of action is broad, we will describe here the most common types of remedies sought and give some examples of how and why they come into play. You will then be able to understand why certain types of director actions yield breach-of-trust lawsuits and what state attorneys general are trying to accomplish by filing these actions.

First, attorneys general have the authority to seek orders from the court to prevent ongoing breaches of trust, usually by requesting a *temporary restraining order* from the court at the time the lawsuit is filed. Such an order usually prohibits the directors and the charity from engaging in certain conduct—that is, it maintains the status quo prior to the alleged breach of trust until the case can be resolved through litigation or settlement. This remedy is used in a wide range of circumstances.

A simple example involves cases of abandonment of trust—what we have referred to previously as violations of the duty of obedience to purpose. This remedy is the primary response to all violations of this duty.

Assume, for example, that your hospital raised substantial funds based on the representation that the money was to be used to build and operate an urgent-care center serving a specific community, and you have now decided that you no longer wish to provide that service. Your board votes to sell the property on which the center is located, cease operations, and use the proceeds for other purposes.

An appropriate response by the state attorney general might be to file an action claiming abandonment of the trust. These facts would support a legal conclusion that the fundraising created a restricted trust requiring those assets to be used for the specific purpose for which they were raised. The attorney general is likely to seek a court order barring your hospital from selling the land and requiring that you continue to use those assets for their required purposes or transfer them to a successor charitable corporation that will honor the trust restriction.

This type of action is usually filed against the board of directors and the charitable corporation. It is a nonmonetary remedy; the goal is to ensure compliance with the trust terms and prevent a breach of trust rather than simply to recover money damages. This action is available to attorneys general in all cases in which there is a present and ongoing threat of a breach of trust.

In an egregious case, this action can be combined with an action to remove the offending directors or trustees and to surcharge them (lawyer-talk for assessing monetary damages against someone). Both of these remedies will be discussed later in this section. This type of relief is also often utilized in cases involving charitable-solicitation fraud and in cases involving illegal self-dealing or commingling of assets.

A second common remedy is a *damage action* to recover charitable assets lost through a breach of trust. This is the type of action that is most distressing to board members, for it almost always names them personally and seeks money damages against them. It can be used by attorneys general whenever there has been a loss of charitable funds as the result of actions, whether negligent or willful, that constitute a breach of trust.

This action causes the most concern and the greatest risk to directors when it involves losses caused through self-dealing or other conflicted transactions. Say, for example, that your hospital has purchased computers from a company owned by one of your board members, and it did so with no competitive bids or other significant inquiry to ensure that the price was the best available. Assume, further, that upon investigation, it is determined that, with reasonable inquiry and effort, the computers could have been purchased for less money from an independent source. What is the likely response of the attorney general?

In California, the response will generally be swift and sure. California Corporations Code § 5233 states that in such instances your board was required to make that inquiry and find the lower price. Having failed to do so and having evidence that the computer deal does not meet the "best deal in town" standard, both the self-dealing board member and the other board members who voted for the deal are likely to find themselves subject to a civil suit for the difference between the sale price and the lowest price the attorney general can prove would have been available. In addition, your D&O carrier is likely to invoke the self-dealing exclusion and deny coverage. Your board is probably conflicted and cannot provide you indemnification. In sum, you are now faced with the likelihood of being sued personally, of being removed from the board, and of having to pay your own legal expenses and any judgment; in addition, you will have caused your friends on the board who authorized the deal to be faced with the same exposure.

This remedy is also common in negligence cases. Suppose your hospital's chief financial officer, in violation of internal policies, invests your entire endowment fund in a speculative oil and gas venture that collapses. A breach-of-trust action for negligence and imprudent investment is the likely response by the state attorney general. That action would first target the chief financial officer and, secondarily, would target any officer or director who was aware of the investment and failed to take reasonable steps to prevent it from occurring. Again, each responsible person will be named as an individual defendant in the lawsuit. It can never be a pleasant experience to see the words "People v. [fill in your name]" on a court document.

In this situation, there is good news on the insurance front. This type of suit is generally covered by D&O insurance. As long as your chief financial officer did not lose more than your policy limits and you kept your insurance current, you will probably suffer only personal embarrassment and not personal financial loss.

A third common remedy is an action for an *accounting and restitution*. The funds of your charity, or the proceeds of your conversion, do not belong to you. It's trust money. Trustees and directors must be able to account for the charitable trust assets placed in their care at all times. If your board fails to take appropriate steps to ensure that all charitable funds are accounted for, the attorney general can seek a court order requiring the charity to render such an accounting. If funds cannot be accounted for, those responsible can be ordered to repay the missing funds.

This remedy is often sought when there has been self-dealing between a director and the charity or a commingling of assets. This remedy is also common when the financial records of a charity are in such disarray that it is impossible to determine where all the money went and who benefited. Because the charity and its board must be able to account for the funds under their control, the burden of proof in such cases is effectively shifted to them. If you cannot show the money was properly used, it is assumed to have been misused, and you will be required to pay restitution to the charity.

This remedy is also available in cases involving violations of the duty of obedience to purpose. Where charitable-trust assets are used for improper purposes, even if not for someone's personal financial benefit, the court may order an accounting concerning those expenditures. If the court finds that improper expenditures have been made, it will order restitution to the charity for all sums misspent, plus interest.

A simple example is the hypothetical diversion of monies from our urgent-care facility. Assume that the property had been sold and the proceeds used to fund other charitable services (educational programs, recreational programs, and so on) in another community. If the court finds that those expenditures violated the express trust that applied to the assets, it will order an accounting and then require that those responsible for approving the improper expenditures (the directors who approved the transaction) pay restitution to reestablish the restricted fund at its appropriate level.

These are easy problems to avoid. If you are in doubt as to the proper manner of using any funds held by your charitable corporation, ask your attorneys for written advice on the issue. If you (or they) are still unsure, you can petition a court for guidance, thereby immunizing your decision from later challenge.

Accounting problems regarding your trust's assets should never arise. Make sure that you have adequate financial systems in place to account for funds. Require periodic financial reports to the board by the chief financial officer. And read the audited financial statements you get on an annual basis, particularly the notes, which often provide clues to problem areas. Remember, this money has been entrusted to you for safekeeping, and you are responsible for it. You are required to be able to show how much was raised, how it was spent, and that all restrictions on its use have been complied with. More important, you are not permitted to commingle charitable funds with personal funds or to fail to keep adequate records. If you violate these rules, both you and your organization will be held financially responsible.

Fourth, *punitive damages* are designed to punish directors for willfully breaching their trust. They are extremely rare and are almost always limited to cases of fraud, self-dealing, or other transactions involving personal profiteering. Like criminal sanctions, they are awarded only in cases of egregious behavior. Your corporation cannot indemnify you for any acts justifying punitive damages either through insurance or contractually. If they are awarded against you, you will pay them yourself.

We will not dwell on this remedy because, in our experience, the only persons ever at risk for such sanctions have intentionally sought to divert charitable funds for their own benefit or have engaged in clearly fraudulent conduct. To obtain this penalty, a prosecutor is required to show either willful misconduct or wanton disregard by the defendant for the consequences of his or her acts. Do not behave in this manner and you will not be at risk.

Fifth, we touched on *removal of directors* earlier, and we revisit that remedy here. When an enforcement agency believes that directors have acted with willful misconduct, have engaged in illegal self-dealing, or have been grossly negligent, they may seek to remove those directors from the board. The court has equitable powers to order this.

This remedy is, in practice, not normally invoked for violations of the duty of care or violations of the duty of obedience to purpose, except in extreme cases. It is, however, commonly sought in cases involving the breach of the duty of loyalty. When directors have engaged in illegal self-dealing or have turned a blind eye to self-dealing by fellow directors, state attorneys general will seek this type of relief. In addition, where the failure to account for charitable assets is significant or where directors have allowed the commingling of charitable funds with personal funds, this remedy is also commonly sought. Although this remedy is nonmonetary, it is particularly embarrassing to directors to have a court order their removal. In the most egregious cases, this remedy is accompanied by a time-limited ban on serving a nonprofit corporation in any capacity.

Because this remedy is normally sought only for willful or other serious misconduct, the simple way to avoid it is to meet your fiduciary obligations.

Finally, *involuntary dissolution of the corporation* is the state attorney general's "neutron bomb" remedy. It is the equivalent of the Internal Revenue Service revocation of tax-exempt status. It is the ultimate punishment of a charitable corporation and is rarely used. The attorney general must file suit to involuntarily dissolve the corporation and must satisfy a court that the only appropriate remedy is to end the corporation's existence. If the attorney general succeeds, any assets remaining will be distributed to a successor charity by the court under the *cy pres* doctrine.

Attorneys general usually seek this drastic remedy only when the charitable corporation has gone so significantly afoul of the law that it is no longer capable of serving a legitimate charitable purpose. In most states, this remedy is statutorily authorized. California Corporations Code § 6511 is an example. Under that code section, the attorney general is authorized to seek the involuntary dissolution on any of the following grounds: "1.) that the corporation has seriously offended against any provision of the statutes regulating charitable organizations; 2.) that the corporation has fraudulently abused or usurped corporate privileges or powers; 3.) that the corporation has violated a law that is grounds for forfeiture of its corporate existence; or 4.) that the corporation has failed to pay its tax liability for five years."

The key point here is that each basis for dissolution involves acts by the corporation itself, not by a single director or group of rogue directors. In these cases, the violations of law can, and should, be punished by sanctions against those individuals personally. This is not a remedy that we normally see imposed on hospitals or other substantial and long-standing charitable organizations. Rather, it is most frequently used against fly-by-night charities set up to scam the public through charitable-solicitation fraud. Nonetheless, you should be aware of its existence.

Internal Revenue Service

For a long time, the Internal Revenue Service had only a single weapon to use in its challenge to breaches of trust: revocation of the tax-exempt status of the charitable corporation. The problem with "all or nothing" options is, of course, that they are rarely used because they are appropriate only in the worst cases. In addition, this weapon was often aimed at the wrong target. When individual directors have misappropriated or diverted charitable funds, the remedy should target them and not the organization, which is the victim. As a result, the Internal Revenue Service was, for the most part, not a significant player in this area.

That changed with the enactment of the "intermediate sanctions" legislation (Internal Revenue Code, § 4958). This statute took effect on September 14, 1995, and applies to both 501(c)(3) and 501(c)(4) organizations. Modeled after the private-foundation rules, intermediate sanctions impose an excise tax on "excess benefit transactions" that involve insiders. In excess benefit transactions the value of the consideration given by the charitable organization exceeds the benefits received by the charity.

This remedy applies only in duty of loyalty cases. It applies only to individuals ("disqualified persons") who, within the five years preceding the transaction, were in a position to exert substantial influence over the affairs of the organization. The taxes are levied on those individuals and on managers who authorize and approve the transaction. The taxes are not levied on the organization itself. These taxes are not insignificant. The first-stage tax is 25 percent of the excess value received by the disqualified person. If not corrected, an additional tax of 200 percent of the excess benefit is assessed. In addition, there is a tax on the organization's managers of 10 percent, up to a maximum of $10,000 per transaction.

Where transactions with insiders are involved, the Internal Revenue Service does not need to prove intent to engage in wrongdoing. This is the most serious provision in the law. The persons involved in the transaction need not have intended to do anything wrong or even to have been aware that a problem existed. If, after the fact, the Internal Revenue Service determines that an excess benefit has been received, a tax liability can be assessed. However, this rule applies only to transactions involving a person who has been in a position to exert substantial influence over the charitable corporation; it does not apply to arms-length third-party transactions.

So, if your charity intends to do a deal with a person who might be within the reach of this law—a common example would be the purchase of a medical practice or joint venture with physicians who sit on your board—we strongly recommend that you consult with tax counsel before proceeding with the transaction.

"Disqualified persons" are not limited to officers, directors, or trustees. Any person who, within the relevant time period, has been in a position to exercise substantial influence over the organization comes within the scope of the law.

The House Ways and Means Committee's report on the bill contained provisions to create a rebuttable presumption of reasonableness for transactions. These provisions may find their way into Internal Revenue Service regulations. To fall under this presumption, the transaction would need to be approved by an independent board of directors or committee thereof under the following terms:

- The board or committee would be composed entirely of individuals unrelated to, and not subject to the control of, the disqualified person.

- The board or committee would have a reasonable basis for its decision (this would normally include having obtained and relied on data of comparable transactions).

- The board or committee would adequately document the basis for its decision (normally this documentation would be included in the minutes).

These taxes have to be paid by the individuals, not by the charitable organization. Attempts to have the charity indemnify the individuals for such taxes may, in themselves, be treated as an excess benefit. Moreover, any such attempt is likely to earn the enmity of the state attorney general's office.

For hospitals, there are a number of potential high-risk areas. Any transactions with physician groups that have substantial influence over the organization are likely to raise red flags, particularly where members of physician groups are on the hospital board. In addition, joint-venture transactions with such groups, particularly where the risks and liabilities assumed by the hospital are disproportionate to the hospital's equity share, are potential problems.

Insider leveraged buyout transactions, common in HMO conversions, would be likely targets of this sanction, as would overly generous compensation packages, severance deals, or retirement deals provided to management as part of the conversion of a hospital.

Our best advice: if your hospital is going to engage in a significant financial transaction with a disqualified person under this statute, obtain competent tax counsel to guide you through the transaction. To do otherwise is to invite serious trouble.

Conclusion

The law in most states gives you tools to avoid personal liability and to ensure that directors and trustees can carry out their responsibilities without assuming unreasonable personal financial risks. Use these tools, and you will not face serious risk of sanctions. If you do not use these tools, the legal penalties can be severe for the individuals involved and the organizations.

So the solution is simple. Avail yourself of the safe harbors and other protections that the law affords. Competent legal counsel should be able to set up systems that take advantage of these rules and protect you. State legislatures have, generally, been sympathetic to the plight of nonprofit directors who volunteer their time and abilities to serve their communities. They have created a fairly broad safety net for normal business decisions, and it makes no sense not to use them.

At the same time, those legislatures have empowered governmental enforcement agencies to safeguard charitable assets. Most agencies take that responsibility seriously. If you violate the laws, and particularly if you do so for your own or another's personal financial benefit, you should expect to be the subject of either a civil suit filed by the state attorney general or a tax penalty imposed by the Internal Revenue Service.

However, if you follow the basic rules set forth in this chapter and work closely with your legal counsel, you should be able to avoid confrontations with the enforcement agencies and serve your charity and community without risk to yourself.

Appendix A:
Glossary

backward-looking valuations—Valuations that are made after a price for an asset has been agreed to by the parties to a transaction and that are used to justify that price.

business judgment rule—The legal doctrine that gives directors of corporations protection against liability for making business decisions affecting the corporation under certain circumstances.

capital calls—Demands for contributions of additional money that a managing partner is allowed to make on the other partners to meet the operating or other needs of the partnership.

careful conduct standard—The rule that excuses directors of corporations from liability for losses that are caused by their decisions if they (1) act in good faith (2) after reasonable inquiry (3) in a manner that the director believes is in the best interests of the corporation, and (4) use the degree of care an ordinarily prudent person would use in a similar situation.

common law—The body of law developed by courts in cases over the years and stemming principally from the law of England.

comparable-companies analysis—A valuation method that looks to the prices of publicly traded companies in the same industry to measure the value of a business being sold.

conditions precedent—Terms of a contract that must be met before the other party is obligated to perform some act.

conversion—Any transaction that results in the transfer of ownership or control of a material amount of the assets of a nonprofit corporation to a for-profit company.

corporate-law standard—The legal standard that applies to the operations of for-profit corporations. This is generally the most permissive standard in that it provides discretion to corporate managers and boards of directors.

cy pres—The court-created doctrine requiring trustees or directors to use charitable assets for purposes as close as possible to those set out in the corporate charter or other document describing the original charitable purposes of the entity when the original purpose becomes impossible or impracticable to carry out.

discounted cash flow (DCF)—A way to value a business by measuring the amount of cash it will generate over a given period of time.

dominant charitable purpose (or dominant charitable purpose test)—The test used by courts to determine permissible expenditures of charitable assets by reviewing corporate documents and the history of charitable expenditures by the corporation.

donative instruments—Documents used to make gifts to charitable organizations (such as wills, trusts, or letters setting forth the terms on which a gift is made).

due diligence—The process of examining the facts necessary to make a reasoned decision about matters of importance to the corporation.

duty of due care—The obligation of directors and trustees of nonprofit corporations to manage the assets under their control with the same degree of care that an ordinary person would use to manage his or her personal assets.

duty of loyalty—The obligation of directors and trustees of nonprofit corporations to avoid taking unfair advantage of their position to profit personally from financial dealings with the corporations.

duty of obedience to charitable purpose—The obligation of directors and trustees of charities to use the charitable assets under their control for the purposes intended by the donors or set out in the entity's governing documents.

express trust—A written instrument creating a trust over specific assets and appointing a trustee to carry out the terms of the trust for its beneficiaries.

fair market value—The most likely price that would be arrived at for the sale of an asset in an open market with both the buyer and the seller being fully informed about all material facts and neither being under any compulsion to sell or buy.

fairness opinion—An opinion by an investment banker or valuation firm that the price received for an asset is "fair" to the seller. It is often expressed in terms of a range of value.

gross negligence—An act that is so unreasonable that it demonstrates a total lack of care.

impressed with a charitable trust—The state of an organization when its assets, whether money or real or personal property, are restricted so that they may be used only to carry out the charitable purposes of the organization.

joinder—The addition of parties to a proceeding or court action.

limited liability company (LLC)—A form of business that gives the owners protection against personal liability for the partnership's debts and liabilities similar to that afforded to shareholders of a corporation.

limited liability partnership (LLP)—A form of partnership that gives the partners protection against personal liability for the partnership's debts and liabilities similar to that afforded to shareholders of a corporation.

limited partnership—A form of partnership in which there are general partners and limited partners. The general partners manage the business and are personally liable for the debts of the partnership. The limited partners have no management powers and are not personally liable for the debts of the partnership. The general and limited partners normally share in the profits of the business.

ordinarily prudent person standard—The rule that requires one to act as an ordinarily prudent person would act in the conduct of his or her affairs.

parens patriae —The English common law doctrine that recognized that the king was the "father of the people" and, therefore, had the power to sue to enforce rights of citizens. In the United States, the *parens patriae* power has been traditionally recognized to belong to state attorneys general.

parity clause—A provision in the articles of a corporation allowing it to do anything necessary to carry out its purposes.

per se illegal—The legal doctrine that makes an act unlawful under all circumstances and for which no explanations are considered by the courts as a defense.

profiteering—Transactions that allow directors or officers of a converting nonprofit to profit personally from the conversion.

put—An agreement giving one party to a joint venture the right to force the other party to buy out its interest in the joint venture.

quasi–*cy pres*—A liberalized version of the *cy pres* rule that allows charitable assets to be used for "substantially similar" purposes rather than for purposes that are "as close as possible" to the original purposes.

quasi-trust-law standard—This hybrid standard, which some states have adopted, regulates the behavior of nonprofit directors. It is generally more liberal that the trust law standard but more strict that the corporate law standard in regulating director conduct.

sanctions—Penalties assessed by a court or the Internal Revenue Service for improper acts by officers, directors, or trustees.

self-dealing—Transactions between a charity and one of its officers or directors that confer some financial benefit on that officer or director.

similar-transaction method—A valuation method that looks to the sale of similar companies in the same industry to measure the value of a business being sold.

simple negligence—An act that is not in accord with the way a reasonably prudent person would act in similar circumstances.

surcharge—Money damages sought against officers, directors, or trustees of nonprofit corporations in enforcement actions brought by regulatory agencies.

trust-law standard—The legal standard that applies to trustees. It is generally the strictest standard in that it limits discretion and prohibits any financial transactions between directors personally and the corporation itself.

value of the consideration—The value of an asset or service that one party to an agreement agrees to give to the other party as payment for carrying out the provisions of the agreement.

Appendix B:
The Law of Fiduciary Duties
Affecting Directors and Trustees
of Nonprofit Hospitals

Trust law imposes three principal duties on fiduciaries of charitable corporations: obedience to charitable purpose, loyalty, and due care. These duties apply to directors and trustees of nonprofit hospital corporations and have special importance in the process of considering conversions. Accordingly, we will discuss the requirements of these duties in the conversion context and highlight the principal legal authorities that are the source of these duties.

Duty of Obedience to Charitable Purpose

Although most discussions of fiduciary duties focus on the duties of loyalty and due care, the duty of obedience to purpose is the fundamental obligation of charitable trustees. What can be more basic than understanding and complying with the specific trust that you are required to carry out? Failure to adhere to your charity's purposes will almost always expose directors and trustees to suit for breach of trust. The Supreme Court of Pennsylvania summarized this duty in the case of *Commonwealth* v. *Barnes Foundation*, 398 Pa. 458 (1960): "What more formidable cause of action could exist than the assertion that the trustees of a charitable trust are failing to carry out the mandate of the indenture under which they operate."

In the case of the sale or joint venture of a nonprofit hospital, this is the threshold issue. You should resolve this issue before all others. It requires the board to answer this question: Can we sell these assets and still comply with our charitable trust?

Defining the Trust

How do you identify the trust? In the case of charitable corporations, the answer is simple—from their articles of incorporation and bylaws; from their donative instruments (lawyer-speak for gift documents); and from their historical uses.

The law is clear in most states that all the assets of a charitable corporation, even those obtained without any specific declaration of the use to which they are to be put, can be used only for the specific charitable purposes described in the articles of incorporation. (*Pacific Home* v. *County of Los Angeles*, 41 Cal. 2d 844 [1953]; *Trustees of Rutgers College in New Jersey* v. *Richman*, 41 N.J. Super. 259 [1956].) This rule applies to any proceeds from a sale, joint venture, or lease of your hospital or health facility. So the first thing you should do when considering whether to convert your hospital is to read the articles and bylaws. They are usually written in plain English, and they will alert you to potential problems that may arise. Failure to review these documents can cause substantial grief for both the hospital and the board members personally.

In a California case, the board of directors of a nonprofit hospital system proposed to convert its hospitals into a for-profit joint venture and to use the proceeds to operate a grant-making foundation. Substantial time, effort, and expense was invested in this project. However, during the regulatory review, it was discovered that the articles of incorporation of the flagship institution stated that "the specific and primary purpose for which the corporation is formed is to acquire and operate a nonprofit charitable hospital and medical center." The articles went on to state that the "corporation shall not, except to an insubstantial degree, engage in any activities or exercise any powers that are not in furtherance of the specific and primary purposes of this corporation." Is operating a grant-making foundation the same as acquiring and operating a nonprofit charitable hospital and medical center? The California attorney general's office felt the answer was obvious—no. It concluded that all the proceeds from the planned conversion attributable to the flagship hospital would have to be used to acquire and operate a similar non-profit hospital and medical center. This course of action was unacceptable to both the buyer and the seller, and, in the end, they abandoned the joint venture.

A similar result occurred in Michigan. Attorney General Frank Kelly's office challenged a "whole-hospital" joint venture between Michigan Affiliated Healthcare System, Inc. (MAHSI) and Columbia-HCA. In that transaction, a for-profit limited partnership would have been formed to which MAHSI would have contributed most of its assets, including the Michigan Capitol Medical Center in Lansing. Columbia-HCA would have served as the managing general partner and would have had day-to-day management responsibilities. Attorney General Kelly filed suit to block the deal, and, in a decision by Judge James Giddings of the Ingraham County Circuit Court, the court declared that the proposed joint venture violated Michigan nonprofit law and MAHSI's corporate charter. The parties abandoned that transaction after the court's decision.

The articles and bylaws are not the only documents that may define the charitable trust on which a nonprofit corporation holds its assets. Donative instruments can also significantly restrict a board's discretion. If your hospital's initial funding (or significant funding for expansion or improvements) came from donations and if those gifts contained specific restrictions, you are bound by them. If you ignore them, your deal may be blocked; a court may remove your board as trustee of those assets; and, in the worst case, a court may surcharge the directors for the expenses incurred, including attorneys fees. (See R. H. Malone, M. T. McEachron, and J. M. Cutler, *The Buck Trial—A Litigator's Perspective*, 21 U.S.F. Law Rev. 585 [1987].)

In a reasonably well-known California case, the *Estate of Beryl Buck*, a woman left approximately $10 million in oil-company stock to benefit "needy" residents of Marin County, an affluent county just north of San Francisco. Ten years later, the stock's value had increased dramatically to more than $400 million. The trustee foundation sought court approval to eliminate the Marin-only restriction and distribute the proceeds throughout the San Francisco Bay area. However, the trustee was unable to show, under the *cy pres* doctrine (explained below), that it was impossible, impracticable, or illegal to comply with the Marin-only restriction. The court denied approval of the proposed change in the terms of the trust. In the end, the trustee resigned in favor of a trustee who would show fidelity to the trust purposes. Although the result of the *Buck* case was harsh, the principle of law involved was one of long-standing precedent. Charities must adhere to the donative restrictions under which they take assets—that is the law! (*St. Joseph's Hospital v. Bennett*, 22 N.E.2d 305 [N.Y. 1939])

Courts also consider the "dominant charitable purpose" of the corporation based on historical operations in determining the trust on which assets are held. Even if your articles of incorporation contain expansive uses—and even if your articles contain a "parity clause" (authorizing the corporation to do any acts in furtherance of its purposes)—courts routinely reject attempts by boards of directors to change the corporate activities if that change would constitute a substantial departure from the historical charitable activities of the corporation.

The leading and most rigid case interpreting this rule is *Queen of Angels Hospital v. Younger*, 66 Cal. App. 3d 359 (1977). Queen of Angels was a Catholic hospital in Los Angeles. Its articles of incorporation contained an express statement of purpose to "establish . . . maintain . . . own . . . and operate a hospital in Los Angeles." Those same articles also included an express statement that it was "to perform and to foster and to support acts of Christian charity particularly among the sick and ailing" and "to house and care for the unprotected indigent sick, aged, and infirm." Finally, the articles contained a parity clause authorizing the corporation to do all acts necessary to carry out these purposes. The corporation had, since its founding, operated a hospital and a medical clinic for the poor within that hospital.

In 1971, the Queen of Angels board decided to lease the hospital to a for-profit hospital chain and to use the lease proceeds to operate a series of outpatient clinics to provide free medical care to the poor and needy in Los Angeles. The board sought court approval for its plan. The Court of Appeals rejected the board's proposal. Adhering strictly to charitable-trust law, the court decided (1) that the dominant purpose of the corporation was to operate a hospital, (2) that Queen of Angels could not abandon its dominant purpose and cease to operate a hospital in favor of operating medical clinics, and (3) that the board of directors of Queen of Angels could either continue to operate a hospital or the court would appoint a successor trustee to operate the hospital. The court of appeals wrote how strict its view of charitable trust law in California is: "This corporation is, however, bound by its articles of incorporation. Queen may maintain a hospital and retain control over its assets or it may abandon the operation of a hospital and lose those assets to the successor distributees—but it cannot do both" (*Queen of Angels* v. *Younger*, 369.)

Many states prohibit charities from changing the dominant charitable purpose that has been established by their articles and historical operations. In *Taylor* v. *Baldwin*, 274 S.W.2d 741 (1952), the Missouri Supreme Court applied the dominant charitable purpose test, although in that case it found that the proposed change did not violate the trust. In *Taylor*, the court approved an affiliation between a community hospital and the Washington University Medical Center. The community hospital intended to sell its existing facility and construct a new hospital facility within the Medical Center. Because both the old and the new operations maintained an ongoing hospital, no change in dominant purpose was found to have occurred. This same dominant charitable purpose test has also been applied in New Jersey and Massachusetts. (*City of Paterson* v.

Paterson General Hospital, 235 A.2d 487 [N.J. 1967]; *Attorney General v. Hahnemann Hospital,* 494 N.E.2d 1011 [Mass. 1986].)

We come to this key point—one whose importance cannot be overstated. Without statutory authorization permitting the sale, lease, or transfer of the assets of a nonprofit hospital (or without prior court-approved modification of the terms of the trust), any court which finds that the dominant purpose of the charitable corporation is to operate a nonprofit hospital will, in all likelihood, reject a conversion that would turn the proceeds over to a grant-making institution. If you do not intend to use the conversion proceeds to operate another nonprofit hospital, the conversion will be barred as a matter of law. And, as in the *Buck* case, your attempt to convert may be argued to be a breach of trust and an abandonment of the trust purposes.

So how can you tell whether you can proceed? Although we are reticent to utter these words, the answer is "ask your lawyer." All states that have adopted the Revised Model Non-Profit Corporation Act probably allow the sale, lease, or transfer of all the assets of the corporation. If your state is among these, conversions are probably permitted, and you may, if you desire, skip directly to the next section about restrictions on the use of proceeds (as the following discussion applies only to states without statutes authorizing such transactions).

If your state law does not contain such a provision, you will need to rely on authorizing language in your articles of incorporation or your state's general corporation law. And, in virtually all cases—particularly if you wish to place the conversion proceeds in a grant-making foundation—you will need to obtain a court order authorizing the conversion. Such a court order will almost surely require a finding that the dominant charitable purpose of your corporation is something other than the operation of a nonprofit hospital. Given the normal incorporation documents of most nonprofit hospitals, this finding will be difficult, if not impossible, to obtain.

Adapting the Trust to Changing Times and Circumstances

When faced with significant financial pressures from managed care and an increasingly competitive health care industry, nonprofit-hospital directors frequently authorize long-term strategic planning to obtain market efficiencies and adjust to changing circumstances. Often, the recommendation that the directors receive is to sell the hospital or to enter into a strategic partnership with a for-profit hospital chain to gain access to capital and increased bargaining power vis-à-vis managed-care organizations. What do you do if, having received such advice, you find that your state law does not authorize conversions and that the articles of incorporation or dominant purposes of your organization require the continued operation of a nonprofit hospital? Fortunately, the law provides an answer. Unfortunately for directors, it is not an easy answer.

The first response we normally hear from directors faced with this situation is "OK, we'll just amend our corporate articles to allow broader uses or to remove the dominant purpose of operating a nonprofit hospital." Although this would be the simplest and easiest solution, normally it will not work. Under the law in most states, such an amendment can alter the trust only on newly acquired assets; all assets obtained under the old articles are impressed with a trust for those "old" purposes. (*Pacific Home* v. *County of Los Angeles*, 41 Cal. 2d 844 [1953].) Directors facing this problem must, therefore, look for a different solution. Although it is a breach of trust for a nonprofit hospital to abandon its trust or to sell its assets below fair market value, directors also violate their fiduciary obligations if they ignore financial realities and allow the hospital that they have been entrusted with managing to deteriorate into financial collapse. Put plainly, the law does not require or allow you to ride the ship to the bottom of the ocean.

The solution is the *cy pres* doctrine. Cy *pres* is the court's ability to permit modification of or deviation from the trust's terms because of changed conditions as long as the proceeds are used in a manner that as closely as possible duplicates the prior charitable purposes. Most states follow this rule of law. Some state legislatures have enacted laws modifying the test under the *cy pres* rule. New York, for example, has a "quasi–*cy pres*" rule that permits corporations to use the sale proceeds for purposes substantially similar to the previous charitable purposes.

Under traditional *cy pres* standards, the courts generally allow changes in the trust terms only if they find one of the following: (1) that continued compliance with the trust is illegal; (2) that continued compliance is impossible; or (3) that because of changed circumstances compliance would substantially impair or defeat the purpose of the trust. The California Court of Appeals has succinctly described the requirements for application of the *cy pres* doctrine as follows: "The power of the court of equity to permit or direct deviation from the terms of the trust is at least as extensive in the case of charitable trusts as it is in the case of private trusts. *The court will direct or permit a deviation from the terms of the trust where compliance is impossible or illegal or where owing to circumstances not known to the settler and not anticipated by him compliance would defeat or substantially impair the accomplishment of the purposes of the trust*" (*Estate of Gilliland*, 44 Cal. App. 3d 32 [1974]; emphasis added).

The third element comes into play in hospital conversions. Do not be misled into thinking that this is an easy test to meet—it is not! Courts are extremely reluctant to permit deviation from the terms of a trust and will always require a strong showing, particularly in cases involving charitable trusts. The California Court of Appeals made this point forcefully in *Stanton v. Wells Fargo Bank*, 150 Cal. App. 2d 763 (1957): "Where the main purpose of the trust is threatened, the courts will and should grant permission to deviate from restrictive administrative provisions. But the court should not permit a deviation simply because the beneficiaries request it where the main purpose of the trust is not threatened and no emergency exists or is threatened."

So, assume that you are a trustee of a nonprofit hospital under the following factual situation:

1. Your state law does not contain an express provision (like that found in the Model Act) permitting you to sell, lease, or transfer your hospital assets.

2. Your hospital's articles of incorporation or donative instruments require that you operate a nonprofit hospital.

3. You are presented with financial projections from management (or independent consultants) that show your hospital to be in an inevitable downward slide of decreasing profitability that threatens financial failure.

The first thing you should do is to determine whether your available options include for-profit strategic partners at all. Remember, to meet the legal requirements for modifying the trust, you will need to show that continued nonprofit status will result in financial failure. If there is another nonprofit hospital that you can merge with and avoid such failure, modification to allow a for-profit strategic partner will almost never be permitted. An exception to this rule may, however, exist in the case of religious hospitals if a showing can be made that a merger with a hospital of a different faith may in itself violate religious principles. Courts are likely to pay deference in this regard. But for secular nonprofit hospitals, the existence of an eligible nonprofit partner whose joinder will eliminate the financial crises will almost always eliminate the for-profit option.

If no nonprofit partner is available, the for-profit option exists in theory. However, proving the case for exercising it is no small task. Mere conjecture based on hypothetical projections of declining profitability with no current financial stress is unlikely to convince a court. As noted by the *Stanton* court: "Certainly, it is true that misguided restrictions . . . should not be permitted to defeat [the] fundamental purpose, but it is equally true that the court should not try to guess what economic conditions may be in a few years by permitting deviations when no real emergency exists or is threatened." You will need convincing financial proof to show that both short-term financial stress and inevitable long-term decline— independent of normal business cycles—exist. You must also show that these trends are the result of structural problems that cannot be avoided under current trust restrictions related to the nonprofit form. If you can show such structural problems, modification of the trust to allow the conversion should be possible.

In sum, if you feel that a change in form is essential to the continued survival of your hospital, take the time and effort to make your case; the court will require it. Our recommendations:

- Retain independent, well-regarded financial consultants to demonstrate a lack of financial viability and to provide strong evidentiary backing for this conclusion.

- Demonstrate the unavailability of an acceptable nonprofit partner.

- Document that you have exhausted all other reasonable options besides conversion.

If you follow these recommendations, you will increase your chances of accomplishing your goals substantially.

Restrictions on the Use of Conversion Proceeds

Assuming that your nonprofit hospital has cleared the conversion hurdle, the next question the board of directors normally faces under the duty of obedience to purpose is, What can we do with the sale proceeds? We will discuss the legal standards that apply to this question in some detail, but two points need to be made immediately.

First, we strongly recommend that you address this issue in your initial preconversion planning, before you make the decision to convert. The reason is simple. Most boards of directors have a fairly firm idea of how they hope to use the conversion proceeds, and a decision to convert is often premised, at least in part, on the ability to implement that idea. It is, therefore, important to know what legal restrictions may apply to the use of those proceeds. It can be a particularly unpleasant turn of events for a board of directors to sign a contract to sell their hospital, close the deal, and then learn that their plan for using the sale proceeds is illegal. They could find themselves with neither their hospital nor the ability to carry out the plan on which the conversion itself was justified. The solution to this problem is fairly simple. Have your lawyers address this issue as part of the preconversion due diligence review. They should give you a clear idea of what your options are and of the best way to meet your goals.

Second, the approaches of state regulatory agencies vary most in this area. Although we will explain shortly the legal standards that should theoretically apply, there is a wide disparity between theory and practice. Generally, the state agency that will review your planned use of the conversion proceeds (which we will call the "charitable-uses plan") is the state attorney general's office, and attorneys general approach this issue in one of three ways. Some states adopt a laissez-faire attitude, essentially giving nonprofit boards broad (if not unlimited) leeway in spending conversion proceeds as they see fit as long as doing so does not result in loss of their tax-exempt status. In such states, conversion proceeds have been used for such disparate purposes as funding concerts and art exhibits, building sports facilities, and even purchasing airplanes to provide youth with flying lessons.

Another group of states take a middle ground, requiring that the conversion proceeds be used for general health care purposes—although this requirement tends in practice to be rather broadly defined to include anything that benefits the general health of the community. Examples of these purposes are nutrition, education, housing, as well as the study of health care trends.

California, however, abides strictly by the trust-law *cy pres* rule. Many would argue that this rule results in poor public policy and that it neither promotes efficiency in providing charitable services nor adequately adjusts to changes in the health care delivery system. This argument is properly addressed to the legislature and the courts, not to law-enforcement agencies. For a detailed and enlightening discussion of the *cy pres* issue, we recommend Professor John G. Simon's article *American Philanthropy and the Buck Trust,* 21 U.S.F. Law Review 641 (1987). Note, however, that there are limits to the legislature's power to "reform" *cy pres* rules. See G. G. Bogert and G. T. Bogert, *The Law of Trusts and Trustees* § 397 (2d ed., St. Paul: West, 1984); *The Trustees of Dartmouth College* v. *Woodward,* 17 U.S. 518 (1819); *Kapiolani Park Pres. Society* v. *Honolulu,* 751 P.2d 1022 (1988); *Dunphy* v. *Commonwealth,* 331 N.E.2d 883 (Mass. 1975).

The *cy pres* rule of law is both clear and unbending. As noted by the California Court of Appeal in the case of *In re Veteran's Industries, Inc.,* 8 Cal. App. 3d 902 (1970): "The words *cy pres* are Norman French for 'as near.' The phrase when expanded to its full implication was '*cy pres comme possible,*' and meant 'as near as possible.' . . . Roughly speaking it is the doctrine that equity will, when a charity is originally or later becomes impossible, inexpedient, or impracticable of fulfillment, substitute another charitable object which is believed to approach the original purpose as closely as possible" (citing Bogert and Bogert, *Trusts and Trustees,* § 431).

Virtually all states recognize the law of *cy pres,* although they apply it in slightly different ways. In states whose attorneys general currently exhibit a laissez-faire attitude toward oversight of conversion proceeds, subsequent office holders with a different philosophy will be able to significantly alter policy with no change in statutory authority simply by vigorously enforcing existing rules of law. Of greater concern to trustees should be the fact that unless the attorney general has affirmatively approved a relatively permissive charitable-uses plan, a successor can challenge the plan retroactively. As a general rule, the defense of laches is not available to contest charitable-trust enforcement actions brought by state attorneys general (*Mosk v. Summerland Spiritualist Society*, 225 Cal. App. 3d 376 [1964]).

What does it mean in practice if your state law recognizes the strict *cy pres* rule and your attorney general follows it? Does it mean that you can use the proceeds only to operate a nonprofit hospital? Usually, the answer is no. Absent an express restriction in your articles of incorporation limiting your purposes solely to the operation of a hospital, you probably have some leeway and a number of options.

Most articles of incorporation contain a fairly broad purposes clause, including phrases that permit "promotion of the general health of the community" or "serving the sick and afflicted" or some other expansive phrase. If you have a clause like those, you should be able to devise a charitable-uses plan that achieves one or more of these goals—with one very significant caveat. The courts can also apply here the dominant charitable purpose test described above. Although you will be permitted to develop a charitable-uses plan that does more than just operate or fund a nonprofit hospital, you will still, under the dominant purpose test, be required to maintain that purpose as your principal activity. Because this model is used in California, it is fairly easy to give you an example of how it works. The California attorney general's office believes that the law has two requirements: (1) that the dominant charitable purpose, providing hospital and related medical care, be maintained in any charitable-uses plan and (2) that the expenditure plan be consistent with the historical pattern of use by the organization.

In practice, these requirements have permitted trustees to choose from three different options. The first option is simply to turn the sale proceeds over to another nonprofit hospital serving the same community. Because this is the closest possible use, the successor charity takes those assets with virtually no restrictions other than those contained in restricted-endowment funds.

The second option involves using the funds to support other nonprofit or governmental hospitals serving the same community, usually through direct grants. This option maintains the dominant charitable purpose while permitting the establishment of a grant-making foundation to administer the conversion proceeds.

The third option permits the existing nonprofit board to retain full control over the sale proceeds, notwithstanding the fact that it no longer operates a nonprofit hospital. Under this option, however, the California attorney general's office requires that a strict plan of distribution be adopted and approved by the court because it feels that the change from an operating charity to a grant-making one is a substantial change in purpose that requires court approval as a modification of trust purposes. Moreover, the subsequent court order establishes the specific terms of the trust and the restrictions on which the conversion proceeds must be held.

In California, two separate approaches have been approved for this third option. The first simply replicates the historical expenditures of the hospital. Categories of patient care are defined, and a charitable-uses plan is developed that requires the expenditure of income at other nonprofit or governmental institutions in direct proportion to historical use patterns. The Riverside Community Hospital used this option when it entered into a joint venture with Columbia-HCA in April 1997, the first transaction approved under California's new law governing hospital conversions. (See J. R. Schwartz and H. C. Horn, Jr., "Deal Makers—Deal Breakers," *Hospitals and Health Networks* [Sept. 5, 1997] for a detailed discussion of the Riverside Community Hospital conversion process.)

A second option, which is perhaps more creative and yet still consistent with the law, involves identifying the "charitable components" of the converted hospital. Essentially the board attempts to distinguish the charitable activities (traditional charity care, community-benefit programs) from the commercial activities of the hospital. The board then creates a series of individual endowment funds with each "charitable purpose" allocated a share of the total equity based on its historical percentage of the total charitable activity.

A prime example of this approach can be found in the case of Good Samaritan Hospital in San Jose, California. In January 1996, Good Samaritan sold its system to Columbia-HCA for $165 million, netting approximately $76 million. Using the charitable-component option, Good Samaritan and the attorney general's office identified three basic components:

- Community-benefit programs (meals on wheels, home assistance programs for frail seniors, community education programs) that had previously been carried out by the hospital

- A school-linked preventive health system that provided care to students in the public schools in the county and that had been operated historically by the hospital

- Traditional charity care for the medically indigent

Expenditures for each of these purposes were determined and averaged over the most recent three-year period. Then three separate endowment funds were established and funded in amounts approximating the historical support each usage had received. This plan was then presented to the Santa Clara Superior Court for approval, and it was approved and implemented.

We need to make one last point about "noncompetition" clauses found in virtually every conversion agreement, whether a sale, joint venture, or lease. Noncompetition provisions normally prohibit the selling charity from engaging in or supporting activities that compete with those of the for-profit acquirer. These provisions may prevent you from complying with your duty of obedience to purpose as viewed either by the attorney general's office or by the court. The last thing you want to do is to sign an agreement containing a noncompetition clause and then find that in order to meet your fiduciary obligations you will be required to violate that agreement.

Examples of this dilemma are easy to imagine. Suppose that your sale agreement prohibits your grant-making foundation from operating or funding any services that compete with the acquirer's for-profit hospital services in the community, but a court finds that the dominant charitable purpose of your organization is to provide non-profit hospital and related medical services in that same community and requires you to spend the sale proceeds on such services. You are now faced with a dilemma: you can either violate the court order—for which you can be held in contempt of court, sanctioned, and removed as trustees—or you can breach the noncompetition clause—for which you will probably be sued by the buyer and then by your attorney general for failing to exercise due care in protecting against this eventuality.

No one should be placed in that position. Fortunately, it is easily avoidable if you anticipate the problem and deal with it during the conversion negotiations. The simplest avoidance method is to put a provision into the conversion agreement that overrides the noncompetition clause should the attorney general or a court mandate a use of the conversion proceeds that would conflict with the noncompetition clause. This approach was used in the Good Samaritan case in California, and we recommend it highly.

Duty of Loyalty

The duty of loyalty is the most important duty for officers, directors, and trustees. The reason is simple. Violations of this duty can have the most direct and personally damaging effects on the individuals involved. If you violate the duty of loyalty, you may face:

- Criminal prosecution, civil damage suits, and tax penalties

- The most aggressive enforcement action by regulatory agencies

- Unpleasant media attention

- The fewest legal defenses

In the worst situations, violations of this duty involve fraud, embezzlement, misappropriation, and diversion of charitable assets. In this appendix, we will not focus on criminal conduct. That conduct is, fortunately, rare and is also almost always intentional. It can easily be avoided—just don't do it! Criminal conduct includes so-called soft diversions of charitable assets, such as using the charity's employees to improve personal property, using corporate equipment and assets in a personal business, or using charitable funds for unauthorized family travel. All these diversions of funds are illegal, and all carry serious penalties. (See California Penal Code, §§ 484, 503; California Corporations Code, § 6811.)

Setting aside criminal conduct, what kind of acts will bring into question the duty of loyalty? The most frequent are those transactions with the charity in which an officer, director, or trustee has a material, personal financial interest. They include classic self-dealing situations, where a director provides goods or services to the corporation for compensation. They include transactions with an independent third-party where, as part of a deal with the charity, the director obtains financial benefits from the third party. Or they can be any other form of transaction where a director uses the trust and confidence of the corporation to obtain a personal financial benefit.

In these situations, directors need to ask the obvious questions: What are the legal rules with respect to the duty of loyalty? What can I do and what is illegal? Unfortunately, the answers to these questions vary significantly from state to state. And although the legal rules do tend to fall into two general categories (the trust-law standard and the corporate-law standard), the differences within these categories are sufficiently important that a general knowledge of the rules will not protect you. For example, although California law follows a quasi-corporate-law standard that permits self-dealing under certain circumstances, a charitable corporation may never lend money to a director without the prior written approval of the attorney general's office (California Corporations Code, § 5236).

The best advice we can give you is that if you are inclined to engage in a self-dealing transaction, ask your lawyer for a written opinion of the legality of the proposed transaction, including a full discussion of the legal standards. Get that opinion before you enter into the transaction, and read the opinion to make sure that you understand it. Although directors are permitted to rely on the opinions of experts under the duty of due care, the trust-law standard under the duty of loyalty allows no exceptions: violations are illegal, no matter who tells you otherwise. In addition, the business judgment rule, which normally protects directors, is not applicable to self-dealing transactions.

General Standards

Having given you this warning, we can provide some background and general rules that will help you understand the basic principles that apply to the duty of loyalty and that will also help you to identify specific transactions that invoke this duty and to understand the reasons why the law regulates them.

English common law recognized that fiduciaries should not use their position for personal financial gain. Nor should they place themselves in a situation that creates a conflict between their interests and those of their beneficiary. The U.S. District Court for the Northern District of California stated the rule succinctly in *People v. Larkin et al.*, 413 F. Supp. 978 (1976), interpreting pre-1980 California law:

A trustee may not use or deal with the trust property for his own profit, or for any other purpose unconnected with the trust, in any manner. . . . He cannot take part in any transaction in which he, or anyone for whom he acts, has an interest present or contingent, adverse to that of his beneficiary. . . . It is against public policy to permit any person occupying fiduciary relations to be placed in such a position that he may be tempted to betray his duty as a trustee. *Hence the rule is unyielding that a trustee shall not under any circumstances be allowed to have any dealings with the trust property, with himself, or acquire any interest therein.* (emphasis added)

This is the trust-law standard, and it constitutes an absolute prohibition against self-dealing. Any transaction between a trustee and the trust is per se illegal. "Good faith" is not a defense. Although this was the predominant view in the past, it is no longer the general rule in the United States. However, it still is the view of the Restatement 2d Trusts (see § 379(b)), and it may be followed, in whole or in part, in states that recognize a fiduciary obligation between directors and charitable corporations.

Most states have moved to a more permissive rule that more closely approximates the corporate standard. Under the corporate standard, the test for a transaction to satisfy the duty of loyalty has three components: disclosure, approval or ratification by a majority of the disinterested board or membership, and fairness to the charity. As we previously noted, there are enough exceptions to this general test to require a detailed examination of the specific standard in every case. When dealing with the duty of loyalty, reliance on rules of general applicability is foolhardy at best. Some of these state-by-state variations are so significant that they deserve, in our view, to be accorded separate categories of their own. The California statute is one example.

Table B.1 summarizes the duty of loyalty rules under three separate standards: the trust-law standard, the corporate-law standard, and the California standard. In the following sections, we discuss each of these standards in detail and provide practical examples of how they work in real-life situations.

Trust-Law Standard

The trust-law standard is the simplest standard. It prohibits all self-dealing transactions between a director and the corporation. The rationale for this rule was articulated by the Wisconsin Supreme Court over one hundred years ago: "Trustees are prohibited from self-dealing with charity property not . . . because they might not in many instances make fair and honest disposition of it to themselves, but because the probability is so great that they would frequently do otherwise, without danger of detection, that the law considers it better policy to prohibit such purchases entirely, than

Table B.1. Loyalty standards

Trust-Law Standard	Corporate-Law Standard	California Standard
Absolute prohibition against self-dealing	Full disclosure of the director's interest in the transaction *and*	Disclosure of interest and approval by a majority of the board members without the votes of interested directors
	Approval by a majority of the disinterested directors or members *or* "Fair" to the corporation	Principally for corporation's benefit "Fair" to the corporation "Best deal in town"

to assume them to be valid except where they can be proved to be fraudulent" (*in re Taylor Orphan Asylum*, 36 Wis. 534 [Wisconsin 1875]).

Federal tax law imposes this rule of law on managers of private foundations (Internal Revenue Code, § 4941), and it is incorporated into some state statutes. (See Arizona Corporation Act of 1933, § 4-33-150(b).) The effect of this strict rule of trust law is to prohibit any inquiry into the motive of the self-dealing trustee. As noted by the *Larkin* court, "Courts will not permit any investigation into the fairness . . . of the transaction, or allow the trustee to show that the dealing was for the best interest of the beneficiary. [Citations omitted.] So strictly is this principle adhered to that no question is allowed to be raised as to the fairness or unfairness of the contract" (978).

The rule is plain. If your state maintains the trust-law standard and you are a director or trustee of a nonprofit corporation, you are absolutely forbidden from engaging in any financial transactions with the organization. If you do so, you will forfeit any profits earned in the transaction to the charitable corporation, and, in the event of any loss or damage to the charity, you will be surcharged for the amount of the loss. You may also be removed as a trustee. Moreover, violations of the trust standard are statutorily denominated a "fraud" on the charity, raising the issue of nondischargeability in bankruptcy. Again, the solution is simple—in states that utilize this standard, do not engage in any self-dealing transactions.

Corporate-Law Standard

As we indicated previously, the corporate-law standard has now become the predominant standard governing the duty of loyalty on the part of nonprofit directors. It is the standard recommended by the American Bar Association Revised Model Non-Profit Corporation Act, and it is the standard currently adopted by most states.

(See, for example, 8 Delaware Corporations, § 144; Arizona Corporations Act, 10-3862; Colorado Non-Profit Corporations Act, 7-128-501 et seq.)

Unlike the trust-law standard, the corporate standard does *not* absolutely prohibit self-dealing transactions. Rather, it allows them subject to specific standards and statutorily established approval procedures. The corporate-law standard for the duty of loyalty was aptly stated by the Delaware Supreme Court in *Cede & Co. and Cinerama v. Technicolor, Inc., et al.* 634 A.2d 345, 361 (1993):

> Corporate officers and directors are not permitted to use their positions of trust and confidence to further their private interests. . . . A public policy, existing through the years, and derived from a profound knowledge of human characteristics and motives, has established a rule that demands of a corporate officer or director, peremptorily and inexorably, the most scrupulous observance of his duty, not only affirmatively to protect the interests of the corporation committed to his charge, but also to refrain from doing anything that would work injury to his corporation, or to deprive it of profit or advantage which his skill and ability might bring to it, or enable it to make in the reasonable and lawful exercise of its powers. The rule that requires an undivided and unselfish loyalty to the corporation demands that there be no conflict between duty and self-interest.

As the Delaware court's language suggests, the standard of loyalty imposed under the corporate rule requires unequivocal fealty to the corporation. In practice, however, this standard is somewhat diluted by the ability of either the board of directors or the members to immunize conduct that might, in truth, fall short of the actual standard.

Under the corporate standard, states generally provide three separate ways in which a self-dealing transaction can be immunized from challenge. The first method is through disinterested board approval. A transaction can be approved under this standard (1) if the terms of the transaction are disclosed to or known by the board and (2) if a majority of the disinterested directors vote in good faith to approve or ratify it. As noted by the court in *Cede*: "The Delaware General Corporation Law . . . Section 144(a)(1) appears to be a legislative mandate that, under such circumstances, an approving vote of a majority of informed and disinterested directors shall remove any taint of director or directors' self-interest in a transaction" (345). Alternatively, for nonprofit corporations with members, an informed and disinterested majority of the members can approve the transaction. Finally, most states permit the self-dealing director to avoid liability by showing that the transaction was "fair" to the corporation. In all such instances, the self-dealing director will have the burden of proof.

Regulators and public-interest advocates complain that in the reasonably clubby world of corporate board rooms, friends and colleagues can often immunize conduct that fails to meet the proper legal standard. However, the law in fact permits such immunization as long as the transaction was entered into in good faith, it was neither collusive nor fraudulent, and the board was provided with all relevant information. "Good faith" is most often defined in this context as "the absence of bad faith." As long as the board members do not conspire with each other, are not aware of contrary information, and do not act in a fraudulent manner toward the corporation, they will be judged to be acting in good faith. It is not a terribly difficult standard to meet (*Gaillard* v. *Natomas Co.*, 208 Cal. App. 3d 1250 [1988]).

For directors thinking about engaging in a self-dealing transaction, disclosure is the key! The greatest risk of liability lies in failing to avail yourself of the protections built into the system. If you neglect to provide your board with all the relevant information with respect to the self-dealing transaction, you may well forfeit the immunity that the ratification or approval provisions of the corporate standard permit.

Two additional caveats also need to be mentioned. First, any other director or member who stands to benefit financially, either directly or indirectly, from the transaction is not disinterested. Even if another director's financial deal is separate and independent from yours, if it arises out of the same transaction, it taints that director and his or her vote cannot be used to absolve you from potential liability (*Cede*).

Second, remember that removing the taint of self-dealing does not mean you are home free. It merely brings the transaction within the business judgment rule under the duty of due care (*Paramount Communications Inc.*, *et al.* v. *QVC*, 637 A.2d 34 [1994]). You must still satisfy the standards of the fiduciary duty of due care, which will be discussed in the next section. And as you will see, these duties continually interrelate.

Therefore, if you intend to engage in a self-dealing transaction in a state that utilizes this standard, take advantage of the law to reduce (but not eliminate) your personal liability exposure:

- Fully disclose all the relevant facts of the transaction to your board and document this disclosure in detail.

- Abstain from participating in the vote on the transaction.

- Make sure that a majority of the disinterested directors receive your disclosure documents and vote to approve your deal.

- Do not collude or otherwise impair the integrity of the voting process; an absence of good faith will negate board ratification or approval.

If you take these steps, the corporate standard generally will protect you.

Most states provide that the attorney general or a court (in a proceeding to which the attorney general is a party) may also preapprove a self-dealing transaction. (See, for example, California Corporations Code, § 5233(d)(1)).) This option provides a board with the greatest degree of protection, but it also provides the greatest risk of disapproval, is the most time consuming, and is the most expensive. For these reasons, it is not frequently used. Note, however, that it does provide directors who choose to use it immunity from future challenges to the transaction. Moreover, in California, even if approval by the attorney general is not sought, the law provides an incentive to give the attorney general notice of the transaction. The statute of limitations for challenges to a self-dealing transaction by the attorney general is reduced from ten years to two years when the attorney general is given the required notice.

California Standard

When the California legislature enacted the new Nonprofit Corporation Law in 1980, it changed the loyalty standard in California from the trust-law standard to a quasi-corporate-law standard. (See California Corporations Code, § 5233.) However, the California rules are substantially stricter than the corporate rules found in most states. In our perhaps parochial view, the California statute provides a useful compromise standard that is less strict and more flexible than trust law but more rigorous than the standard for for-profit corporate boards.

The California standard establishes a four-part test that must be passed for all such transactions, and each part must be supported by sufficient evidence to defend the explicit findings the statute requires the board to make. The four parts of the test:

1. The corporation entered into the transaction for its own benefit (California Corporations Code, § 5233(d)(2)(A)).

2. The transaction was fair and reasonable for the corporation at the time it was entered into (California Corporations Code, § 5233(d)(2)(B)).

3. The board's approval was given in good faith, with knowledge of the material facts of the transaction and of the director's interest, and by a majority of the board members currently sitting without counting the votes of any interested directors (California Corporations Code, § 5233(d)(2)(C)).

4. Prior to authorizing the transaction, the board determined after reasonable investigation that the corporation could not have obtained a more advantageous deal given the circumstances (California Corporations Code, § 5233(d)(2)(D)).

Only after all four tests have been passed can a board properly authorize or ratify a self-dealing transaction under California law.

A close look at this standard demonstrates that it provides significantly greater protection for the charitable corporation than does the general corporate standard. First, it requires approval by a majority of the existing board, not just a majority of the disinterested board members. Although interested board members can be counted to determine whether a quorum of the board is present, their votes cannot be used to obtain a majority. (California Corporations Code, § 5233(g).) This rule is crucial where a majority of the board is conflicted, as is the case in some insider leveraged buyouts. In those cases, under California law, board ratification is not available, and approval would have to be sought either from the court or from the attorney general using the procedure we outlined earlier.

Second, the California law requires that the corporation enter into the transaction for its own benefit. This means that the board must determine that the transaction is necessary for the corporation independent of the interested director's desire to have the deal.

Third, the California standard requires a finding of fairness in addition to, not in lieu of, board approval. Thus, the board making a fairness finding and approving the transaction is at risk should a court later determine that it was wrong.

Finally, and most important, the California law requires the board to be able to satisfy what we call "the best deal in town" provision. This provision provides the greatest protection for the charitable corporation. It requires the directors to conduct a reasonable inquiry to determine whether the corporation could have obtained a more advantageous deal from another party and, if so, requires the corporation to get no less favorable a deal from the self-dealing director. In our view, this provision almost always requires the board to identify alternative transaction partners, request pricing data, document this information, and disclose it in full to the board. In complex large transactions, like conversions of HMOs or hospitals, it will virtually always require a market-bid procedure because there is no other effective way to determine that the transaction could not be effected on more advantageous terms.

In this regard, we often see "fairness opinions" from investment-banking firms or valuation firms that appear designed to meet the general corporate standard. In the conversion of nonprofit hospitals, these opinions usually rely substantially on the discounted-cash-flow methodology. Our experience indicates that although these opinions may be sufficient under the general corporate standard, they will almost never meet the California "best deal in town" test. The reason is simple: these opinions do not purport to represent the most likely market price for the assets, let alone the most advantageous one. Rather, they appear to measure the investment value of the asset to the seller. These are two different standards, and, in fact, it is not uncommon for the market price for a hospital to be twice the discounted-cash-flow value. Failure to determine and obtain the "best deal in town" disqualifies a self-dealing transaction from board approval in those states applying California's standard.

California Corporations Code § 5233(h) gives judges significant discretion in awarding damages for self-dealing transactions that violate the law. The court may do any of the following:

- Order all profits from the transaction returned to the corporation.

- Order the self-dealing director to pay the corporation for all benefits received.

- Order the return or replacement of the property or assets involved, including lost income and appreciation.

- Order an accounting of the financial transaction.

- Order the board or the self-dealing director to pay prejudgment interest and punitive damages.

The court is also required to take into account factors that mitigate the need for damages, including benefits received by the corporation and the good faith of the self-dealing director.

In sum, the California standard provides, as many legal commentators have recommended, a middle ground between the trust and corporate standards. And because the California statute was used as the basis for the Revised Model Non-Profit Corporations Act, it may signal an evolving national standard.

Real-Life Examples

How do these varying standards work in the real world? We will provide two typical situations and then apply the standards. We will, of course, not discuss the trust-law standard because no such transactions are permitted under that strict rule.

The first example involves the sale of an HMO to its management team, including ten of the fifteen board members. The corporation has no members. Under the general corporate-law standard, the self-dealing directors can attend the board meeting and their presence would constitute a quorum. Then, after full disclosure to the five disinterested board members, three of those disinterested directors can vote to approve the transaction. Their vote would constitute valid approval, effectively immunizing the transaction from attack under the duty of loyalty. Those three disinterested directors would have to act in good faith, but if they did so the transaction would pass muster.

But remember that the duties of loyalty and due care are interrelated. Therefore, this approval brings the transaction within the business judgment rule. However, in transactions that involve a breakup of the corporate entity or a change in control of the corporation, the general corporate standard may now impose an additional duty to obtain the best value—a standard analogous to the California "best deal in town" test. This is the rule espoused by the Delaware Supreme Court in *Paramount Communications, Inc., et al. v. QVC*, 637 A.2d 34 (1994). There the court decided that "[t]he consequences of a sale of control impose special obligations on the directors of the corporation. In particular, they have the obligation of acting reasonably to seek the transaction offering the best value reasonably available." (See also *Barkan v. Amsted Indus.*, 567 A.2d 1286 [1989].)

Thus, in our example, the directors' vote to approve the buyout would have removed the taint of self-dealing under Delaware's duty-of-loyalty standard and brought them within the business judgment rule. However, they would still need to meet the enhanced test of proving that they obtained the best price under their duty of care.

How would this transaction fare under California law? The answer is, procedurally quite differently, but substantively much the same. The key procedural difference is that under California law there are not enough disinterested directors to approve the transaction. Therefore, to meet the requirements of § 5233 and obtain the benefits it provides, the directors would have to either seek the approval of the attorney general or obtain court approval in a proceeding in which the attorney general was a party.

These are tests that both the attorney general and the court would apply:

- Was the transaction done to benefit the corporation?

- Was the transaction fair to the corporation when entered into?

- Was the deal the "best deal in town"?

Failure to pass these tests would subject the directors to the damage provisions of § 5233(h) discussed above.

At the risk of being too clever, we have used an example in which the substantive standards that are ultimately applied are the same under both rules—essentially the "best deal in town" test. We have used this example because conversions involving insider leveraged buyouts have been quite common in the health care industry. However, this particular result occurred only because our hypothetical example involved the sale of the entire corporation. Had it involved the sale of only some of the corporate assets, the lesser corporate standard would have simply applied a good-faith and rationality test under the business judgment rule.

Our second example involves the sale of a hospital-owned MSO to a physician group where two of the physician-group members serve on the hospital's ten-member board of directors. Under the corporate-law standard, again assuming that the sale was approved by a majority of the disinterested board members, the transaction would be required to meet only the business judgment rule. The board would have to show that it acted in good faith, that it felt the transaction was in the corporation's interest, and that its decision was rational.

California law would, in this instance, require a far more stringent showing. The hospital board would be required to make reasonable inquiry and then make a formal determination that all the § 5233 standards that we previously discussed had been met, including the "best deal in town" test. Also, the "intermediate sanctions" rules under the Internal Revenue Code would come into play in this example, and they are of significant importance.

Duty of Due Care

The duty of care is just what its name implies—an obligation to be sufficiently careful in making decisions that involve charitable assets to protect those assets from loss. A court enforcing this duty will look at the decision-making process used by a board of directors to determine whether the board members did an adequate job of informing themselves of the facts. It is, in effect, a due diligence test. Because the duty of care comes into play in almost every decision a director makes, you must understand the legal requirements that it imposes.

The simple truth is that none of us is perfect. Sooner or later a decision made by your board is going to turn out badly for your nonprofit corporation, whether it's a hospital, skilled-nursing facility, university, or foundation, and money will be lost as a result. An understanding of this duty will give you the necessary tools to protect yourself from personal liability for those losses.

To understand this duty, you need to focus on (1) the legal standard of care imposed in your state and (2) the procedures that your state permits you to follow to minimize your liability exposure. In this section, we will discuss both these issues in detail.

Although this duty interrelates with the duty of loyalty, we will assume for the purposes of this discussion that the transactions involved do not involve self-dealing or other conflicts of interest. As you now know, such conflicts cause the more stringent duty-of-loyalty rules to be applied.

We also need to alert you to one additional, and very significant, fact. This is an area in which there is a significant discrepancy between legal theory and legal practice. Courts in different states, claiming to invoke the same legal standards and using the same legal terms, impose different rules. For example, most legal commentators say that the business judgment rule protects directors against negligence claims and permits liability only for gross negligence. However, numerous court decisions claiming to invoke the business judgment rule have imposed liability for actions that look very much like simple negligence. (For our purposes, *simple negligence* is generally defined as the lack of ordinary care, and *gross negligence* is defined as an extreme departure from ordinary care or a conscious disregard or entire failure to exercise care.)

Therefore, although we will explain the theoretical legal rules in sufficient detail for you to be generally familiar with them, we will focus most of our discussion on the standards actually applied by the courts, regardless of the terms used to describe them. In this way, you will understand what is expected of you under the duty of care. From there, we will go on to discuss the specific procedures you can employ to protect yourself from liability under this fiduciary duty.

Standard of Care

Frequently legal commentators will claim that the difference in the standards of care found in the various states depends largely on whether an individual state applies a trust-law or a corporate-law standard of care. However, we are not aware of any state that holds directors to a "pure" trust-law standard with respect to the duty of care. Rather, the difference in state standards depends largely on two factors: whether a state includes within its rules an "ordinarily prudent person" standard and how its courts interpret this standard. Those states that apply the ordinarily prudent person standard in a literal way bring their law within what is commonly called the "careful conduct standard." Although this standard tends to require a somewhat greater showing than simple negligence to impose liability on directors, it does not require the far more stringent showing of gross negligence or willful misconduct. (See *Burt v. Irvine Company*, 237 Cal. App. 2d 828 [1965]; *McDonnell v. American Leduc Petroleum Ltd.*, 491 F.2d 380 [1974]; and *Johnson v. Johnson*, 515 A.2d 255 [New Jersey 1986].)

Those states that do not include this language (or whose courts are unwilling to interpret it literally) generally apply a corporate business judgment rule that permits liability only for gross negligence or bad faith. (See *Beard* v. *Achenbach Memorial Hospital,* 170 F.2d 859 [Kansas 1948]; and *Cede & Co. and Cinerama* v. *Technicolor.*)

Table B.2 compares the differing elements of these two legal tests. You should begin any discussion of your duties by identifying which standard applies to you.

When attempting to determine the applicable standard of care, you need to be aware, first, that although almost every state has enacted a general nonprofit corporation law, only about one-quarter have included an express statement of the applicable standard of care for directors. The majority of states rely on court decisions to establish the rules. In those states that have created specific statutory standards exclusively for nonprofit corporations, almost all use

Table B.2. Standards of care

Business Judgment Rule[a]	Careful Conduct Rule[b]
1. Good faith and without a conflict of interest	1. Good faith
2. A conscious decision made on a reasonably informed basis	2. After reasonable inquiry
3. With a rational belief that the business judgment is in the best interest of the corporation	3. In a manner the director believes is in the best interest of the corporation
	4. With such care as an ordinarily prudent person in a like situation would use

[a]See American Law Institute, 1 *Principles of Corporate Governance: Analysis and Recommendations* (1994).
[b]See California Corporations Code, § 5231.

the careful conduct standard. (See, for example, California Corporations Code, § 5231; New York Not for Profit Law, § 717; Minnesota Statutes 317.20(6); and Connecticut General Statutes 33-447(d).) This is also the standard recommended by the Revised Model Non-Profit Corporations Act.

Second, states that apply the business judgment rule do so differently. The Delaware Supreme Court highlighted this fact in the *Cede* case. There, the Delaware court noted that in a previous case, *Graham v. Allis Chalmers Mfg. Co.*, 188 A.2d 125 (1963), the court had used the prudent person standard in implementing the business judgment rule. The *Cede* court criticized the prudent person standard because it "appear[s] to protect only director actions that do not constitute simple negligence." The court noted that Delaware courts historically applied the business judgment rule to immunize "all director action not constituting gross negligence." (See *Aronson v. Lewis*, 473 A.2d 805 [1984]; *Smith v. Van Gorkam*, 488 A.2d 858 [1982].) California courts interpreting the business judgment rule have also used language that appears to create something akin to a simple-negligence standard. In *Burt v. Irvine Company*, the court decided that directors who "commit an error of judgment through . . . want of ordinary prudence and skill may [be held]. . . responsible for the consequences" (852).

How then are you to know what the rules are in your state? The answer is that this is no game for amateurs—ask your lawyer! We will, however, attempt to explain these standards as they are enforced in the real world so that you can get a reasonably clear idea of how they differ in practice.

The Standards in Practice: Good Faith, Reasonable Inquiry, Due Diligence

Good faith is the key to avoiding personal liability. Both the business judgment rule and the careful conduct standard incorporate a good-faith requirement. In practical terms, this means that you must ensure that all your decisions avoid conflicts of interest. Once again, there is a significant difference in how this requirement is implemented under the two standards. Under the business judgment rule, full disclosure to the board of directors of the material terms of the transaction and of any conflict, accompanied by the approval of a majority of the disinterested board members, cures the conflict problem and satisfies the good-faith requirement. The transaction will satisfy the duty of care if it meets the remaining tests listed in Table B.2.

But the transaction will not satisfy the duty of care under the careful conduct rule and certainly not under the California version of it. The existence of a conflict of interest that is covered by the self-dealing rules requires the application of the self-dealing standard alone. Therefore, once it is determined that the self-dealing rules apply, that statutory standard and not the due care standard applies. For example, under California law a director who self-deals will always be judged under the strict duty-of-loyalty standards found in Corporations Code § 5233, not under § 5231. But, in most states, the general corporate business judgment rule allows approval by a majority of disinterested board members after full disclosure to satisfy the good-faith requirement.

Both standards require directors to obtain the information necessary to allow them to make an informed decision. In this regard, the standards are not dissimilar. California courts, using the reasonable-inquiry standard have concluded that "directors may not close their eyes to what is going on about them in corporate business, and must in appropriate circumstances make such reasonable inquiry as an ordinarily prudent person under similar circumstances." (*Gaillard* v. *Natomas Co.*, 208 Cal. App. 2d 1250 [1989].) Similarly, the Delaware Supreme Court decided in *Cede* that this component of the business judgment rule "requires a director, before voting on a proposed merger or sale, to inform himself and his fellow directors of all material information that is reasonably available to them."

This is not a new rule. In 1913, the Oregon Supreme Court ruled in *Devlin* v. *Moore*, 130, p. 35, that "[i]f nothing has come to knowledge to awaken suspicion that something is going wrong, ordinary attention to the affairs of the institution is sufficient. If, on the other hand, directors know, or by exercise of ordinary care should have known, any facts which would awaken suspicion and put a prudent man on his guard . . . want of that care makes them responsible."

What does this mean in practice? First, as a director, you must make the effort to obtain the facts necessary to make an informed decision. If you do not read the materials provided to you before you vote on an issue, courts are unlikely to believe that your vote was reasonably informed. If your managers do not provide you with adequate information to make a reasoned decision and you rubber-stamp their conclusions without getting sufficient information, courts are unlikely to believe that your vote was reasonably informed. And if you are aware, or should be aware, of significant problems with a transaction and do not seek the information necessary to fully evaluate those problems, a court is unlikely to believe that your vote was reasonably informed.

Second, the greater the significance of the transaction, the more likely the courts are going to be to impose stringent standards of inquiry on directors both to obtain all relevant information and to obtain independent professional advice. This is already the law in the state of Delaware. In *Paramount v. QVC*, the Delaware Supreme Court ruled that in decisions involving the sale or transfer of control of a company, "special obligations" are imposed on the directors of the company, and "the courts will apply enhanced scrutiny to ensure that directors have acted reasonably" (43).

The logic of this ruling is inescapable and equally applicable to nonprofit corporations. What decision can be more important than one to abandon the ongoing charitable operations of a nonprofit corporation and turn it into a grant-making foundation? Therefore, in cases involving the conversion of nonprofit institutions, we think it likely that the courts will always require a rigorous investigation of all relevant issues. In particular, we believe it is doubtful that with respect to issues like valuation and analysis of operating agreements in joint ventures, a board of directors will ever be in compliance with this requirement unless they have retained knowledgeable independent experts to review these matters and advise them appropriately. If you fail to take these steps, you are, in our view, inviting a challenge on due diligence grounds.

How is the due diligence standard applied in real life? As the *Cede* court rightly stated, the ordinarily prudent person standard is essentially a simple-negligence test. Because we have previously noted that this is the standard recommended by the Model Act and may, therefore, become the national standard over time, certain obvious questions come to mind. Are directors in states that have adopted this language liable on a showing of simple negligence? Are they liable even if that same state has recognized and applied the business judgment rule to nonprofit corporations? Fortunately, the rules are not as severe as one might fear.

Again, California law serves as a useful example. California has adopted the ordinarily prudent person standard for both for-profit and nonprofit corporations. (See California Corporations Code, § 309 (for-profit) and § 5231 (nonprofit).) California has also applied the business judgment rule to both for-profit and nonprofit corporate directors. (See *Gaillard* v. *Natomas* [for-profit] and *Lee* v. *Interinsurance Exchange*, 50 Cal. App. 4th 694 [1996, nonprofit].) However, California law marries these two concepts in what we think is a logical and workable way, with an emphasis on process. Liability is not predicated on a failure to make a "good" or a "correct" business decision in every case. That would place an undue burden on directors and dissuade even the most dedicated from serving. Rather, the directors' obligation is to conduct that level of inquiry necessary to justify the making of the decision. And the more important the decision, the greater the required level of inquiry. Thus, the decision of how much information is needed before reaching a conclusion is reviewed on something approaching a simple-negligence standard. Did the board conduct the inquiry that would be engaged in by an ordinarily prudent person in like circumstances?

However, once this process standard is met, directors are generally immune from liability for their decision provided it is within their discretion under the corporation's internal rules and is not entirely irrational. As such, the business judgment rule does not conflict with the due care standard, it complements it. An articulate statement of this principle was made by the court in *Burt* v. *Irvine*, 237 Cal. App. 2d 828:

> A reconciliation of these two concepts is found in *Casey* v. *Woodruff* [citation deleted], wherein it is stated: "The question is frequently asked, how does the operation of the so-called 'business judgment rule' tie in with the concept of negligence. There is no conflict between the two. When courts say that they will not interfere in matters of business judgment, it is presupposed that judgment— reasonable diligence—has in fact been exercised. A director cannot close his eyes to what is going on about him in the conduct of the business of the corporation and have it said that he is exercising business judgment. Courts have properly decided to give directors a wide latitude in the management of the affairs of the corporation provided always that judgment, and that means an honest, unbiased judgment, is reasonably exercised by them."

The New Jersey courts have reached similar conclusions. (See *Johnson* v. *Johnson*, 515 A.2d 255 [1986], holding that New Jersey's prudent person rule is consistent with the business judgment rule.)

It is our view that this standard is not that difficult to meet. It requires directors to obtain a sufficient amount of information to inform themselves prior to making corporate decisions, and the greater the importance of the decision, the greater the level of required inquiry. Once this inquiry is complete, however, the business judgment rule will protect virtually any rational decision.

·And because the law in most states permits the delegation of the information-gathering process and reliance on those selected to do it, no director should ever be faced, in our opinion, with a challenge under the duty of due care. Almost every potential problem can be avoided by a process that is focused on providing a firm basis for decision making.

Process Protections

Now that you are alarmed by the widely varying statutory standards and misleading legal rules that govern your conduct, you may ask yourself, How can we be so confident that almost all potential pitfalls under the duty of care can be easily avoided? The answer is that process cures almost everything. Keep in mind that the duty of care is process-oriented. The courts will look not at the wisdom of the decision itself so much as at the decision-making process that was used. If you create a proper process, you can virtually immunize your ultimate decision regardless of how badly things turn out.

In a California case, a nonprofit hospital corporation decided to create an integrated delivery system, enter the managed-care business, and expand its operations significantly. It lost tens of millions of dollars. Understandably, it also drew the attention of (and audit by) the California attorney general's office. After an exhaustive inquiry, the attorney general determined that the hospital directors had carefully considered each step before taking it, had obtained competent expert advice for each decision and relied on it in making their decision, and had kept themselves informed about the economic problems and taken reasonable steps to deal with them on an ongoing basis. In hindsight, one could certainly question the wisdom of those decisions, but that is not the legal test. Each decision was made in good faith, after due diligence, and with expert advice—all that is necessary to satisfy the legal tests for the duty of care. As a result, the attorney general's office closed its investigation and informed the board that its decisions fell within the protections of the business judgment rule.

Conversely, if a board decides to invest its endowment fund in speculative ventures and does so (1) without adequate investigation of all material facts, (2) without receiving expert advice, and (3) without a full analysis of the risks and rewards involved, any loss of assets will surely make the board vulnerable to a breach-of-trust lawsuit based on the duty of due care.

These two examples demonstrate that although the legal standards with respect to the duty of care vary widely in different states, the procedural requirements to immunize board decisions from challenge under this duty are quite similar. This is true regardless of whether a particular state imposes the careful conduct standard or the corporate business judgment rule. Therefore, you have no excuse for failing to follow legally permissible procedures that will protect you and your board.

How do you create a process that provides the maximum protection? You make sure that you do two things well: (1) delegate responsibility and (2) rely in good faith on the information and advice you receive.

Virtually all states authorize board members to delegate the task of conducting due diligence to corporate officers and managers, to outside experts and consultants, including counsel, and to committees of the board on which they do not serve. (See New York Not for Profit Law, § 717; California Corporations Code, § 5231.) Therefore, it is never an excuse to say, "We didn't have the time to conduct a sufficient inquiry and obtain the information necessary to make an informed decision." If your entire board lacks the time or expertise to conduct a due diligence inquiry, then delegate that responsibility to those who do.

But keep in mind a warning. Give those to whom you delegate this responsibility adequate time and adequate resources to do the job properly. If you do not, two problems may arise. First, a lack of adequate time and resources in the delegation can bring into question the good faith of the board in making the delegation. Second, you can expose those management personnel or retained experts to potential negligence or malpractice lawsuits for failing to do an adequate job.

So, if you are going to avail yourselves of this option, do it properly. Engage competent persons to do the inquiry. Give them adequate time and resources to do the job. Make sure your board minutes accurately reflect the decision to delegate responsibility in this regard and that a complete and thorough review was requested. Absent some egregious shortcoming in the delegation decision itself, this process should immunize your board from liability exposure for this part of the process.

Not surprisingly, the law in virtually all states permits directors (once they have delegated responsibility as discussed above) to rely on the information they receive. So our advice to directors is to take advantage of these provisions in the law. Have those to whom the delegation of due diligence is made provide written reports to the board detailing their efforts; consider those reports carefully; document that consideration and reliance in the board minutes; and then take the appropriate action.

Although these steps will generally protect you from liability exposure, there are two significant exceptions. First, although your board has the right to rely on those to whom the delegation was made, you are not permitted to ignore information of which you are aware (or should be aware) that runs counter to these recommendations and that puts you on notice of problems in either the due diligence process or the recommendations received. Virtually all state laws that expressly permit such delegations contain this limitation. New York law is a good example; § 717 of the Not For Profit Law provides that "[p]ersons shall not be considered to be acting in good faith if they have knowledge concerning the matter in question that would cause such reliance to be unwarranted."

Second, any conflict of interest on the part of a director (in a state using the careful conduct standard) or undisclosed and unapproved conflict (in a state using the general business judgment rule) will destroy the protections provided by these procedural steps.

In addition, in the area of hospital conversions, there is increasing concern over the delegation of due diligence responsibility to senior management. In a great many instances, those managers are conflicted by personal self-interest in the transaction because of their desire to remain in place at the converted hospital, often with much higher compensation. However, boards of directors typically rely on their chief executive officers and chief financial officers in these areas. This reliance creates an inherent weakness in the credibility of both the advice received by the board and the board's decision, which is necessarily based in large part on that advice.

One possible solution to this problem is California's legislation in this area. Senate Bill 413 recognizes this inherent conflict and deals with it in a measured way. Those members of senior management who are unwilling to disqualify themselves from post-conversion employment with the buyer may still provide advice to the board. However, the board may not "substantially" rely on that information and advice without having it vetted by an independent expert. Failure to comply with this mandate violates the standard of due care under the statute. The law does, however, provide the directors with a safe harbor. If they retain an independent expert to confirm the information and advice received from potentially conflicted managers, they are deemed to have complied with the statute. This approach permits the board to receive input from its senior management while, at the same time, providing protection against potential conflicts. Boards considering conversion transactions should seriously consider implementing some version of the procedures mandated in California to ensure that their process is not infected by serious conflicts of interest.

Index